EFFECTIVE MANAGEMENT OF PRIVATE HEALTH CARE

Editors: Anthony Byrne and Haydn Cook

EFFECTIVE MANAGEMENT OF PRIVATE HEALTH CARE

Edited by: Anthony Byrne, Chief Executive of
the Independent Hospitals Association and
Haydn Cook, Director of Parkside and
Hillside Hospitals

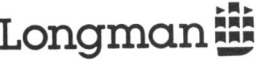

Longman Group UK Limited
Longman House, Burnt Mill, Harlow, Essex, CM20 2JE

© Longman Group UK Limited 1989

First published 1989

British Library Cataloguing in Publication Data

Effective management of private health care.
   1. Great Britain. Private health services. Management.
   I. Byrne, Anthony   II. Cook, Haydn
   362.1

ISBN 0-582-04283-6

Typeset by Next Step
Printed and bound in Great Britain by Bell & Bain, Glasgow

Editors' foreword

The private sector has now come of age. This book is a celebration of that maturity.

Discussions between Longman and the Independent Hospitals Association last year suggested a need for a book covering various aspects of private health care management. The chapter writers bravely volunteered their services. We are all practical managers rather than professional writers and so putting down in words a description of our actual practices has not been easy.

The editors and writers welcome comments, and would be pleased to be involved in discussions with readers. This book is an attempt to express a first view and will, it is hoped, be refined in further editions.

All contributors have asked us to state that their views are their own, and not necessarily those of their employers. The editors have tried to avoid making substantial changes to contributions, and each chapter is therefore very much a reflection of each writer's perspective of health care.

In a way it is a privileged insight into a private world. Many business sector managers are obsessively secretive about their businesses, and their approach. Our chapter writers are leading exponents: their confidence in their ability to keep one step ahead means that they are willing to share with you the secrets of their present success.

As editors we should like to thank Alan Dearling of Longman for his help and support. We thank the contributors, all of whom work in a high pressure environment, and we know that making time to write meant making sacrifices in many ways. Thanks also to Tim Battle, Unit General Manager of St Stephens and Westminster, Ron Kerr of the Department of Health, Linda Satchell of The Lister, Chelsea Bridge, and one editor would especially thank Meriel Cook.

Anthony Byrne
Haydn Cook

The editors:

Anthony Byrne is Chief Executive of the Independent Hospitals Association.

Haydn Cook is Hospital Director, Parkside/Hillside Hospitals, and Board Member of Paracelsus UK.

Contents

Introduction

Good managers are hard to find. In our relatively young independent health care industry we have no long historical tradition to illuminate 'the way we do things here'. Rather, each manager seeks to apply sound management principles in his or her own organisation or hospital.

In this book the chapter authors contribute to a valuable forum of information exchange. They each illustrate a major aspect of management specifically for the independent health-care sector. In doing so they exhibit a professional attitude and a concern for high standards of patient care which are typical of the sector.

The book will be invaluable for both existing and aspiring managers in independent hospitals and homes. It will provide an equally useful insight for NHS managers who are grappling with the new problems of marketing and competition in the health service.

Alan M Dexter
Chairman
Independent Hospitals Association

Alan Dexter is Chief Executive of Community Hospitals.

Contributors

John Cassell	Director Strategic Healthcare Associates
John Jackson	Corporate Director of Operation AMI Healthcare
John Rigby Jones	Finance Director Great Northern Hospitals
Sally Taber	Director of Nursing London Bridge Hospital St Martins Hospitals
Robin Scott	Director of Recruitment Services Catalysis Ltd Principal Taylor Scott Associates
Sandra Hallett	Management Consultant
Paul Ridout	Solicitor
Ben Thomas	Director BUPA Occupational Health
Haydn Cook	Hospital Director Parkside/Hillside Hospitals Paracelsus UK
Peter Naylor	Chairman Catalysis Ltd

1 Marketing

John Cassell

Modern organisations recognise that a customer orientation is crucial. Hospitals must concentrate on providing those services and facilities which their customers want of them. As an organisation, a hospital must constantly look outwards to see what the market wants and to monitor what the competition is doing. We therefore felt it appropriate to begin with a chapter on marketing.

History

Although many people have suggested that marketing started with Adam Smith, serious application of marketing principles came in the early fifties when companies such as General Electric became marketing led in a traditional production driven industry.

Service industries adopted marketing at a much later date and in the UK health care marketing did not begin formally until the early eighties in the private sector. The NHS, post Griffiths, has now started to show interest in marketing and the strong themes of competition and customer responsiveness in the recent White Paper will undoubtedly push health authorities towards marketing their services.

Ethical role

A key area of resistance to marketing has come from its clash with the vocational aspect of health care particularly amongst the nursing and medical professions. Marketing is associated with hard selling, special offers and gimmicks that are in stark contrast to patient care delivery. This type of misunderstanding about the role of marketing is still common in the UK and when driven by competitive pressure to 'do some marketing', mangers will often ask their secretaries to invite the local editor for lunch, or will have an open day once a year. These 'soft' manifestations are designed not to offend the managers' professional colleagues. The true relevance of marketing in the health care environment however, comes in a much broader setting. In the words of Philip Kotler:

> *Marketing is the analysis, planning, implementation and control of carefully formulated programmes designed to bring about voluntary exchanges of values with target markets for the purpose of achieving organisational objectives. It relies heavily on designing the organisation's offering in terms of the target market's needs and desires and using effective pricing, communication and distribution to inform, motivate and service the markets.* (Kotler and Clarke, 1987)

It is clear that a 'voluntary exchange of values' and responding to the target markets' needs and desires is more concerned with matching the organisation's capabilities with customer needs than forcing the customer to accept what he does not want. Thus in this wider sense, the marketing of health care services can sit comfortably alongside its ethical tradition and should be a method whereby customer service is enhanced.

Marketing orientation

There is no well established traditional role for marketing in health care delivery and many organisations taking it up, assign duties often of a limited nature to a staff person who is called on where necessary.

In progressing towards a true marketing orientation, McDevitt (1987) in a US study, identified four stages of development that hospitals go through in achieving a marketing orientation:

- *Inside-out marketing*
  At this stage the needs of the hospital rather than the customer are met and the attitude is that the management know best. There is rarely a marketing person and little attempt is made to understand the customer.

- *Promotional marketing*
  Generally consists of promoting services the management have decided they should provide. Research into the effectiveness of services, delivery or service promotion may be undertaken.

- *Integrated tactical marketing*
  At this stage the facility recognises its role in fulfilling customer needs and within the limits of its overall plans will attempt to achieve this. Marketing personnel will be recruited and a full range of tactical marketing initiatives will be undertaken.

- *Outside-in marketing*
  This final stage sees a market orientation being introduced to the overall strategy of the hospital. A true external marketing perspective is developed by analysing customer needs at an early stage and applying that knowledge to strategy development. Typically there is a full application of marketing techniques and importantly an understanding and participation in the role of marketing throughout the organisation.

In the UK, the majority of organisations are at the 'promotional marketing' stage and very few have moved through to the last two stages. This situation is changing rapidly however and a number of factors are causing increased interest:

1 More competition and better knowledge of what to expect amongst doctors and patients, who now choose with authority.

2 Reimbursement pressures and cost escalation that has frequently increased the occupancy required to break even.

3 The recognition that the profitability of different patient groups can vary significantly and that the overall performance of a facility can be improved by selectively concentrating on certain segments.

4 Pressure from groups of hospitals or other facilities taking patients through Preferred Provider or similar exclusive arrangements with insurers, local authorities or other patient sources.

5 Recognition that utilisation of resources is not influenced effectively on a day-to-day basis and that some planned programme is needed to ensure regular activity for the staff, equipment and accommodation which are a permanent and expensive feature of health-care facilities.

There are thus significant pressures on modern managers, be they in charge of an alcohol rehabilitation unit in the country or a high technology acute care hospital in town. They may be faced with declining occupancy. They may have a major disaster with the Press on the telephone every hour. They may simply not know where the next patient is coming from. All these problems can only be addressed effectively by the correct application of marketing principles.

Responsibility for marketing

Compared with their NHS or overseas counterparts most health care facilities in the UK private sector are small. Acute hospitals for example average only fifty beds.

The inevitable question is whether a marketing professional can be afforded on a full time basis. The classic compromise is to give 'marketing' to someone in the organisation as an additional job or to take on someone with limited experience.

Bearing in mind the lack of marketing development, selling marketing to the rest of the staff and doing it, is too much for one person and turnover of marketing executives has been very high. More success has been achieved by recognising that since health care succeeds or fails on the quality of the people delivering it, then each employee is part of the marketing effort of the organisation. Thus when the person in charge also provides the marketing leadership and direction then the whole organisation will become market responsive.

Table 1.1 Specialist marketing skills

Function	Resource
Market planning	Preferably in-house and part of the overall business plan. Can be facilitated by outside agencies
Market intelligence	Managed in-house but outside agencies can provide data sources
Market research	Basic studies, i.e. doctor interviews, in-room questionnaires etc. can be carried out in-house. More complex research should be briefed into a research agency
Pricing and reimbursement planning	In-house jointly by marketing and finance
Advertising	Brief with outside agency for both promotional and recruitment to ensure consistent quality of image
Direct mail	Brief into outside agency
Literature, publications in-room information etc.	Brief into outside design/copywriting agency. Print can often be purchased in-house
New product/service feasibilies	Preferably in-house between relevant department, marketing and finance
Public relations	Trained in-house resources may be supported by outside agency
Sales	Trained in-house resource, external sales training

Many hospital directors now have formal marketing backgrounds and the marketing manager route is considered a valid line of progression to general management.

Clearly this is not going to provide the whole marketing resource solution. It does, however, allow for the additional marketing functions in the hospital to be of a specialist nature or bought in from the outside.

Table 1.1 gives the major specialist marketing skills and typical resources for a health care facility. From this it can be seen that the marketing executive needs still to have all-round skills and can act as a resource for the rest of the organisation in the areas of market research, advertising, and most particularly, creating an appreciation of how well the facility is performing in its market-place.

1 EXECUTIVE SUMMARY

2 SITUATION ANALYSIS
   • Environment and assumptions
   • Performance
   • Strengths, weaknesses, opportunities and threats analysis (SWOT)

3 MISSION STATEMENT AND CORPORATE GOALS

4 MARKETING OBJECTIVES AND STRATEGIES

5 MARKETING ACTION PLANS

6 PERFORMANCE EVALUATION AND CONTROL SYSTEM

Figure 1.1 Marketing plan structure

Marketing plan

The marketing plan is the method by which the organisation manages its profitable growth and with the operational and financial plans makes up the overall annual business plan for the facility. Too many times the annual budget is developed simply as an acceptable percentage activity increase on the previous year and the marketing manager is then asked to find some programmes to make it happen. This wastes the opportunity to take a much firmer grip on what is possible for the business by using the market planning process.

There are many ways of approaching market planning and as with other management disciplines it is better to start off with a system that the organisation is comfortable with and increase its sophistication over time as the process finds acceptance. The process outlined in Fig. 1.1 covers the basic action steps necessary. The process should be led by the marketing manager or in his or her absence by the director of the facility but should involve as many of the key staff as possible. This adds to the marketing awareness overall and gains commitment to the key action plans that will often depend on a large group of the work force for their successful execution.

Executive summary

This should be a concise statement of the salient features of the plan that will aid communication with a number of interested audiences including: senior management; medical or community boards; heads of departments.

Situation analysis

This section may simply be developed as a part of the marketing plan but is extremely important in determining the overall objectives for the facility, for operational and financial planning. Thus while it is addressed here, in an ideal world most of the data will be collected on an ongoing basis throughout the year and reviewed in its broadest sense at the beginning of the planning cycle.

It is often valuable to use the situation analysis as one component of a pre-budget retreat where an overview of the strategic direction of the organisation can be developed as a backdrop to the planning process. The retreat can also emphasise the essentially market driven rather than internally driven approach that is necessary for good planning.

There are three main components to the situation analysis: environment and assumptions; performance; SWOT.

Environment and assumptions

Included under this heading would be those general external factors that have an influence on the performance of the facility. Rather than collect every available statistic in sight as a surrogate for real understanding, it is better to concentrate on those where a clear connection with performance can be established. Typically these might include:

1 Major demographic changes, e.g. significant growth in population of the elderly or of white collar high-tech work-forces.

2 Movements in the insured population, e.g. overall 5 per cent increase, but 2 per cent increase in company paid market.

3 Changes in unemployment level by industry where, for example, shortages of skilled labour might cause an increase in the employee benefits offered.

Overall statistical trends often hide opportunities amongst focused sub-groups, and it is worth spending time at this stage of the plan looking behind the figures. Some assumptions also need to be made and documented as to the future trend of these environmental factors.

With a number of conflicting influences such as interest rates, local economy, health legislation, etc., there is a reluctance to make firm predictions on environmental trends. Unless this step is taken, however, later strategy decisions become more tenuous.

Performance

The main performance statistics gathered by health care organisations tend to be primarily functional and often only those specifically responding to statutory business requirements.

From the marketing perspective, these are important, but must be supplemented with additional information to give an overall view of how well the facility is satisfying market opportunities.

Figure 1.2 lists some typical performance information for an acute-

Population data
- Size of the catchment area (by post code)
- Population in the catchment area (preferably by post code)
- Numbers, ages, sex, socioeconomic groups, social groups, income levels, insurance cover
- Mix of patients using the hospital, market shares, out migration from the catchment area

Medical services data
- Doctors in the catchment area
- Consultant locations, specialities, ages, NHS hospital base
- Users/non-users/multiple hospital users: activity levels by location
- GP locations, special interests, size of practice, private practice
- Referral pattern by hospital/consultant

National Health Service Facilities
- Locations of hospitals, number of beds, principal specialities, pay beds, pay-bed occupancy/revenue
- Waiting lists by specialty, revenue generation activity, contracting activity, technology base: excess capacity/shortages

Competition
Comparative analysis of all competing hospitals assessing parent company capabilities (if relevant); image/community awareness; staff/management performance; activity levels and market shares by specialty; doctor base/location; financial performance; technology base; pricing policy; insurance coverage; comparative service delivery performance

Insurance base
Hospital market share of insured population in the area by major insurer, policy and patient source, i.e. company paid, voluntary group or private payment

Industry
Industrial base in the area by SIC code, number of employees and health insurance cover

Hospital performance
Three-year activity trends covering:
- financial - revenue, profit before tax, capital expenditure, ROI, ROCE;
- utilisation - admissions, average length of stay, outpatient visits, day cases, performance by specialty, performance by consultant user, performance by insured/uninsured mix;
- other revenue generating activity - overseas patients, outpatient programmes, health screening/occupational health, consulting rooms, NHS contracting, etc.;
- image/community awareness - research results;
- quality performance indicators - research results.

Figure 1.2 Performance information for an acute-care hospital

care hospital. This is not exhaustive and will vary with each type of facility. The value of all information needs to be critically reviewed, bearing in mind that data collection often involves major expense.

Competitor studies is an area in which accurate data are hard to come by, although with staff moving from one competitor to another, there is more competitor knowledge in the organisation than first meets the eye.

If we recognise that the marketing objectives a facility finally agrees upon are in opposition to a similar set of marketing objectives in the competition, then our chances of success are weighted heavily by our insight into our neighbour's likely strategy.

SWOT

This acronym representing an analysis of strengths, weaknesses, opportunities and threats has become a common method of generating an overview of a facility's position in its market place.

It is best developed using a group of managers with additional perspectives being provided by members of medical staff or associated community representatives. Sheila Edwards (unpublished), in Fig. 1.3 sets out the typical general subjects that might be covered by a SWOT analysis in a hospital setting.

The mission statement and corporate goals

The marketing plan has to be consistent with the overall purpose and direction of the organisation, therefore, part of the input into plan development should include the current mission statement and those corporate goals that are relevant to the marketing activity.

Not everyone has a mission statement and this may lead to confusion amongst staff as to the true purpose of the facility. The exercise of developing a mission statement often creates some healthy debate and a consistent sense of direction at the end.

The following example of a recently developed mission statement for the Devonshire Hospital in Central London clearly defines a focus of activity in terms of service and customers.

The Devonshire, as a private hospital, provides a highly developed, innovative and multi-disciplinary rehabilitation service to consultants for their UK and international patients.

Corporate goals may specify, amongst others, financial performance criteria for all or parts of the facility, the quality standards expected of service delivery and even the expected role as employer in the local community.

The role of marketing within all of these areas need to be incorporated in the marketing objectives and strategies.

Developing marketing objectives and strategies

Early marketing plans in private health care consisted of a number of generally unmeasurable tactical actions to try and increase awareness or

---

Strengths of hospital
   Nursing staff calibre
   Leading cardiac surgeons associated with hospital
   High quality equipment, e.g. CT scanner
   Larger referral base from GPs

Weaknesses
   Not enough theatre space at specific times
   Insufficient equipment in a specialty
   Not enough interpreters
   No obstetric department
   Limited access by public transport
   No car parking facilities
   Costs of services perceived as too expensive

Opportunities
   Competitor closing wards for refurbishment
   Developing more volume in a specific specialty
   Developing new services which competitors (NHS or private) do not
      have
   Evaluating NHS contract work
   Day surgery units
   Company contracts
   Developing health screening

Threats
   New private hospital opening; NHS improving services
   Consultant fee increases
   Low public awareness of hospital within the community
   Competitor purchasing new equipment - how will it impact on existing
      business?
   Retirement of top user consultant
   Competitor's lower cost of service
   Consultants moving to competitor

Figure 1.3 SWOT analysis

utilisation. The short timescale and apparent ineffectiveness of these plans made them prey to being the first budget cut when performance declined. Logic argues that when fewer customers use your services, you should increase your marketing activity and spend more, but with little knowledge of what worked or why, budget reductions were the usual course of action.

Thus whilst the situation analysis may seem an enormous effort in order to decide on a few marketing actions, it, in fact, substantiates the selection of objectives and strategies and may be needed in some cases to support the spending of large sums of money on the launch of a new product or service. It also enables some sophistication to be introduced in the setting of marketing objectives.

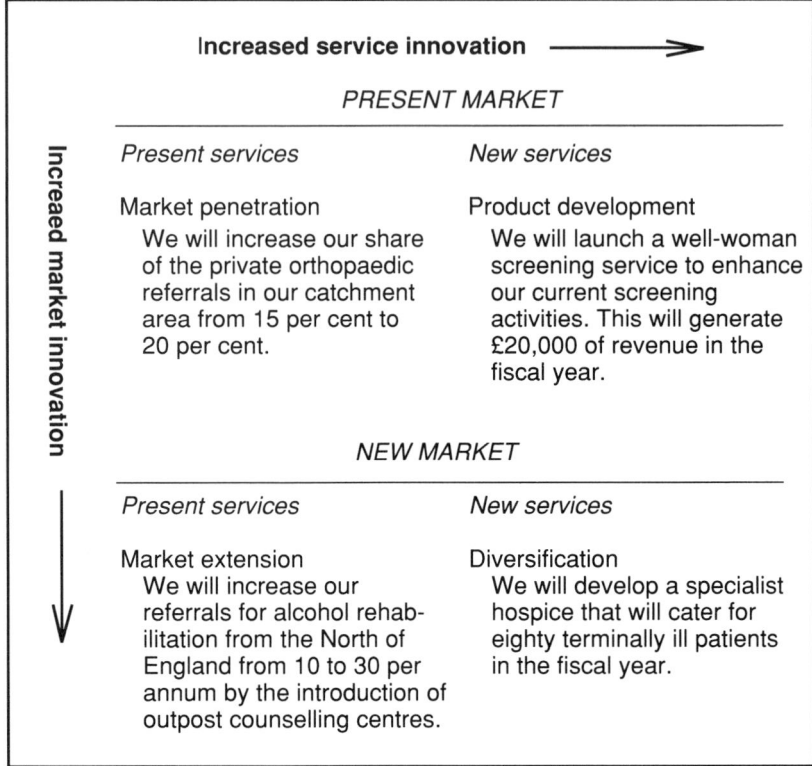

Figure 1.4 Ansoff matrix

In the private health care market, typically, marketing objectives will be designed to build on some already partially developed situation, as the locations of facilities are fixed and the primary markets around them remain relatively constant.

Ansoff (1957) has identified four broad categories of business opportunity and some typical objectives related to these are illustrated in Fig. 1.4.

Segmentation

Marketing objectives state what the organisation wants to achieve and marketing strategies are the method of achieving the objectives. A typical marketing objective for a nursing home might be:

> *To ensure that occupancy does not fall below 80 per cent on average throughout the year.*

It may be that within the nursing home, certain types of patient in terms of their ailment, socio-economic group or simply disposable income, are more profitable or more readily available. Some understanding of these segments of the market can be gleaned from the situation analysis and a more differentiated strategy developed that may, for example, increase revenue by concentrating on couples who are mobile or some other specific group.

Building expertise in delivering service to a specific segment and understanding the needs of that segment better than the competition are excellent ways of protecting your own market. It is unusual for a facility taking an undifferentiated approach to have such a good reputation in a general sense that some parts of its empire are not vulnerable to attack from a competitor attacking a particular segment. The NHS, for example, usually pursues an undifferentiated approach and has lost certain groups of people who have opted for the private sector. However, within the NHS, units such as the Royal Marsden, which have concentrated on a particular specialty, attract patients back from the private sector because of their reputation.

Examples of concentrated segmentation in the private sector are:

Facility	Segment
AMI Portland Hospital	Women and children
Broadway Lodge	Alcohol and substance abuse
Manor House Hospital	Members of the Industrial Orthopaedic Society

The Portland Hospital in London has developed a very strong reputation in obstetrics by a combination of superior service delivery and technology. Thus a newcomer to the London obstetrics market would need to find some specific advantages over the Portland and might well choose another part of the country or another service to offer which would provide an easier entry.

Particularly in competitive situations, therefore, the marketing objectives should look to respond to specific segments.

Understanding the buying decision

Marketing objectives are frequently directed at groups that do not make the buying decision. A current example that will have increasing relevance in the United Kingdom is the desire of health care facilities in the United States to promote their facilities directly to the general public. With more and more hospital selection decisions being made by employers rather than employees, the public's unbounded enthusiasm for a particular hospital may well go unrequited if their employer decides otherwise.

The buying decision often involves a number of players and their degree of influence may alter with time. For a patient to go into a private hospital, some or all of the following will be involved: the patient, the patient's family, the general practitioner, the employer, the consultant and the insurer.

Developing marketing strategies

We find in the private sector that frequently services provided are very similar; a hernia operation is a hernia operation to the unfamiliar patient.

Equally, as we have discussed, a number of different players are involved in enabling the patient to have his hernia operation.

Strategies, the methods by which objectives are achieved, therefore need to be well focused to ensure that yours is the service chosen by the customer.

Using research

Merely selecting a particular segment, i.e. females 18+, as a target for well-woman screening, may not be enough when there are several other suppliers in the vicinity. A detailed understanding of the attitudes of potential service users is necessary, and this may only be achieved by commissioning research. The research may give guidance on a number of factors that will affect success or failure with our health screening product. These can include: levels of interest and attitudes towards cost for different age groups, product modifications to attract 18-25 year old young women versus 60+ elderly women, which groups are best approached through their employer, what media various groups of women read, what style of literature, direct mail or advertising should be used, how many women would have the strongest interest in well-woman screening and where they are likely to live.

Research can create a detailed level of understanding that maximises the impact of a particular strategy, yet it is used infrequently in the private sector other than by health insurance companies. The credibility of marketing activity and the level of success of marketing strategies will undoubtedly increase as more companies recognise the need to invest in research.

Marketing strategy components

The situation analysis, the marketing objectives and associated research enable clear marketing strategies to be developed. These are conveniently divided into a number of products or services, and their associated pricing, policy, promotion or distribution.

If we go back to our well-woman screening example, following the research we may have decided to target young women between 18 and 25 and have discovered that the main benefit sought is prevention of cervical cancer and that there is interest in being associated with other women of a similar age.

The service can, therefore, be designed to emphasise the cervical screening role as opposed to coronary heart disease screening, for example, which is less significant for young women. We may also consider providing the service on certain days of the week and associate it with other services for women of this age, including weight reduction classes, advice on contraception, etc.

A proportion of the target market may be paid for by their employers, but a larger group will be paying out of their own pockets. For the latter group, the pricing of the service has to be at a level where it has preference over other competing costs, such as entertainment, clothes or holidays, as well as any competitor services. This, again, can be tested by research.

The promotion of our well-woman service will be on a number of levels. Well-woman is a generic description, and we will probably want to brand the service to differentiate it from competitors. This may or may not include the name of the company, depending on whether the company name adds value or confusion. Branding can then be used on all promotional activity to create awareness and choice.

Videos, literature and other printed material can be branded and identified for the target market. For those women paying for themselves, whose readership habits are known, we can consider targeted advertising or direct mail, press articles or special offers in appropriate magazines, and even telephone sales if we have a good sense of where they are likely to be living. The group who may use the service via their company need to be treated very differently, and direct selling activity targeted to the personnel officers of companies with large female work-forces would be more appropriate.

Distribution of the well-woman screen will also vary with the two groups of women. The self-pay group will typically be happy to come to a hospital or clinic. The company-pay group may well be allowed the service only if the screen is brought to the company location to minimise absence from work.

This example provides merely a surface examination of how strategies are developed and targeted to meet marketing objectives. As competition increases in the United Kingdom, more and more sophisticated methods are being employed to ensure that strategies achieve an essential 'closeness to the customer'.

Marketing action plans

The achievement of each strategy is ensured by the development of a series of detailed action plans that cover the day-to-day activity throughout the plan period. A convenient way of laying out action plans is to list them under a main strategy heading, specifying the following criteria: timing, executive responsible, budget, and measurement of success. In this manner, there will be little ambiguity as to what needs to be achieved. The budget for each action can then be incorporated into the total marketing budget and the latter reviewed for cost effectiveness against the anticipated growth of the business.

Thus in the process of moving from overall objectives through strategies into action plans, the routine activities of marketing are focused back to the broad direction selected for the facility. The example in Fig. 1.5 illustrates how this can work for our health screening objective.

Performance evaluation and control system

In an industry dominated by financial control systems, marketing is generally seen as an area almost impossible to measure in terms of its

---

Marketing Objective Example
  We will launch a well-woman screening service to enhance our current screening activities. This will generate £20,000 of revenue in the first year.

Marketing Strategy Example
  We will contract with at least two industrial companies to provide well-woman screening at the work place by running a series of screening presentations to company personnel officers.

Action Plan Example
  Well-woman screening presentations

Timing	Executive responsible	Budget	Measurement of success
September and November	Marketing manager/ Screening doctor	£600	100 well-woman screens

---

Figure 1.5 Relationship between objectives, strategies and action plans

effectiveness. It is easy to determine, for example, the catering costs per patient per day, but less so the outpatient revenue resulting from a particular advertising campaign.

Undoubtedly, most tactical marketing programmes take place in a changing environment and often have multiple effects, but it remains essential to tie down as accurately as possible the results generated from each pound of marketing spent, including personnel costs, as well as promotional or other expenditure.

Many companies have advertised in their local market for years, yet have retained no record of media performance. As much information can be gained from advertising failure as advertising success, and it is relatively straightforward to pay attention to response rates from different creative approaches, different publications, different types of advertisement, different positioning within the publication, advertisements with and without coupons, advertisements with editorial, frequency of insertion, etc.

Often the view is that 'advertising does not work for us', whereas by looking back over past failures, it may be that a certain creative approach with a coupon inserted fortnightly on the television page of the local newspaper actually works extremely well.

The performance of programmes that on the face of it do not have any strict measurement criteria can often be evaluated by broader studies, such as research into the awareness of the facility in the community, or as part of researching patients or doctors.

The amount of effort put into this part of the marketing activity pays dividends, both in terms of more cost-effective results and defensibility of the marketing plan when it has to compete with other departments for budgets each year.

Marketing audit

We have seen that whilst there may be specific executives responsible for the bulk of the marketing activity, almost everyone in the organisation participates in marketing in one form or another.

Therefore, even the chief executive who officially 'doesn't do' marketing probably would be surprised by the amount of hidden cost that is associated with marketing activity.

Marketing audits are a method of evaluating the appropriate focus and effectiveness of marketing activity throughout the organisation. Audits should be carried out regularly to an agreed format that questions all aspects of marketing activity, and are ideally led by someone who is independent of the function; an internal auditor, for example, would be very suitable.

Each audit should be developed specifically for the organisation involved, but will generally cover the relative performance of the organisation in the following areas: the market-place in general; the competition; and the elements of strategy, i.e. service delivery, pricing, promotion, distribution.

Marketing information system

For both the situation analysis and for evaluating marketing programmes, it is important to maintain a method of gathering marketing data. The most interesting information that is gathered from a marketing point of view will be the trend in some activity, e.g. referrals from a segment of the population, the impact of pricing changes on volume, etc.

The marketing information system, like the recording of financial trends, should provide both regular and *ad hoc* reports on key indicators of performance and factors that impact the facility in general.

There are two primary sources of information for the marketing information system: internal data, i.e. trends in occupancy, referral patterns, length of stay, etc.; and external data, i.e. trends in population, competitors, medical practice, etc.

These are augmented where necessary by market research that will provide specific information not readily available, such as customer satisfaction levels or attitudes to new services. Computer models and other more advanced techniques can also help quick evaluation of the impact of certain trends on the organisation.

Overall, the marketing information system is designed to improve the quality of marketing decision making, and its development is often, unfortunately, prompted by the discovery of some disastrous trend that has not surfaced in the normal financial analysis.

Service in marketing

Health care marketing differs from many other forms of marketing in the very importance of the people delivering the service. There are tangible things that customers or patients have opinions on, e.g. hotel services, information provided, even staff uniforms, but the difference is primarily made by the hands-on interaction with doctors or staff. Thus a critical part of the health care marketing function is internal marketing to the staff. Staff, just as patients or doctors, become another customer to satisfy on the basis that their satisfaction and understanding of what the organisation requires of them, are reflected in good service to the doctor and patient.

There should be, either within the marketing plan or perhaps as part of the training or personnel function, a series of actions to ensure that internal marketing is being addressed, e.g. employee satisfaction research, customer satisfaction research and feedback to staff, effective communication of general company and marketing objectives and strategies, devices for suggestions and ideas to flow back from staff to management, etc.

These and other similar programmes are often as significant as external marketing activity in shaping the performance of the organisation.

Summary and future trends

This brief overview has indicated that in a few years the marketing function has become recognised as an essential part of the management process in the private sector. The approaches used remain fairly basic, at this stage, but pressures from competition, cost escalation and reimbursement control are accelerating interest in this field. The wealth of knowledge in the industry is being augmented by the appointment of more marketing professionals and more general managers with marketing backgrounds.

The increased comfort with the timescales involved in marketing, as opposed to day-to-day operational issues has led to a greater awareness of long term trends that influence the business.

Facilities that have been extremely successful for many years have found their markets being eroded by long term trends that inevitably caught up with them, and the traditional life cycle of launch, maturity and decline has been found to apply to some well-established institutions.

To predict and plan for this changing environment, there will be a greater interest in developing strategic plans at both the facility and group level. Capital expenditure, particularly in the for-profit end of the industry, is increasingly justified by detailed feasibilities, which, again, are best seen in the context of an overall strategic plan.

This trend and the market orientation it brings will help to ensure that in the future the marketing plan will become as accepted and commonplace as the revenue budget in private health care.

References

Ansoff H I 1957 Strategies for diversification. *Harvard Business Review* Sept./Oct.

Edwards S (unpublished) *Strategic planning manager* AMI Healthcare

Kotler P, Clarke RN 1987 *Marketing for health care organisations.* Prentice-Hall

McDevitt P 1987 Learning by doing: strategic marketing management in hospitals. *Health Care Management Review* **12**(1): 23-30

2 Management

John Jackson

Having discussed marketing, we move to the question of delivering those services and facilities that customers require. Management is never an end in itself, but rather it is a way of determining targets, and a means of achieving those targets. This chapter addresses those issues, and provides an insight into the skills required.

Basic principles

'Most private patients in Britain today must balance convenience, flexibility and intimacy against safety, technical and medical excellence and comprehensive care.' (Higgins, 1988). The size and scale of activity of an independent hospital are relevant to this. There are problems of scale particularly in the levels of expertise that can be attracted, retained and maintained. With an insufficient workload of certain specialties, say neurosurgery or intensive care, the professional skills of staff in a hospital can soon deteriorate and their loss of motivation will probably lead to a speedy departure. Investment in clinical equipment may be decided upon the financial return instead of the potential clinical need. In these circumstances the actions of an independent hospital must always be ruled by clinical safety for patients.

The National Health Service has undergone many agonies as to what is the optimum size for an efficient hospital: from the massive district general hospitals to the concept of 'small is beautiful'. Independent hospitals are obviously smaller — the range for acute hospitals is from 15 to 256 beds with an average of 50 beds per hospital.

Although the size of some of these independent hospitals has been limited by the potential market for private work at the time of building, this has nevertheless proved to be one of the strengths of those hospitals. Namely they are able to provide an intimate service for patients maintaining that close 'personal touch' that so many patients seek. It also means that there is more flexibility amongst staff, communication is easier, there is a different working relationship with doctors, and other benefits do accrue.

The growth of private medicine is bringing a greater range of clinical services into the independent sector as hospitals generally increase in size and are seeking to complement to a greater extent the services available within the NHS. The potential stimulus from the outcomes of the 1989 White Paper will probably increase that trend in many areas. Given the correct political and financial circumstances some of the largest hospitals within the UK could, and some have, become major players in the provision of health care in their particular communities.

There are some differences in management required between the public and the private sectors that go beyond the issues of scale. Marketing skills which used to be solely in the domain of the private sector are now needed much more within the NHS. Business skills, again an essential tool for survival in the private sector, have developed dramatically within the NHS over the last few years. The great strength of the NHS in its training capability has spread into the private sector with the removal of political ideology and an increased awareness of the value that each party can have for the other. Greater sharing of physical resources in terms of equipment, staff, space or time has helped to a small degree in removing some of the old barriers between the two sectors.

These all lead to a point where the management skills required within either sector — or elsewhere — are similar in many respects and I shall endeavour to highlight some of those skills that are necessary for success in health care. Some of the issues, particularly finance and marketing, are dealt with elsewhere in this book. I refer therefore to these subjects in outline while seeking to describe the necessary skills.

I have been consistently approached by members of staff over the years saying that they wished to learn more about management. When asked to be more specific, in the majority of instances the response was 'well, just general management'. Perhaps this emphasises just one of the problems when writing about management. There are many definitions of management, but for me, in general it is the application of common sense to achieve success in one's particular environment. What are the definitions of success and environment? These will vary from person to person and organisation to organisation.

It is important to recognise that such things as financial and marketing skills are an integral part of management but the most pervasive issue of all has to be the *commitment to quality*. It does not matter whether one is making widgets, building a space shuttle or providing health care — that overall emphasis on quality must exist in every member of the organisation irrespective of their role. This dedication to quality is one of the additional challenges for the manager and unless he or she has it and can communicate it, failure will inevitably follow. I will pick up the issue of quality later.

At this point I will mention my other major principle of management which, like that commitment to quality, pervades everything: *keep it simple.*

I have attended too many conferences and listened to too many presentations on topics that have made the whole situation far too complex. By trying to look at every detail and every issue it is easy to obscure the outcomes that one needs or desires by making a situation too complex. Businesses have failed and battles have been lost because those seeking to control events became too bound up with the apparent complexities and over-abundance of information, too much analysis and perhaps a subsequent reluctance to act in the appropriate manner at the appropriate time. 'Paralysis by analysis' is a popular aphorism. Only by keeping all matters simple, by concentrating upon the opportunities and the threats in relation to one's own strengths and weaknesses, and by being absolutely clear about the desired outcomes, will success follow. That simplicity has to apply to all levels of our health care activities: at the strategic end — the long term future of our hospitals and our businesses; and at the sharp end — the way in which for example each and every patient is received or the way in which goods are purchased. This is not to ignore the fact that hospitals are very complex organisations requiring the co-ordination of many diverse activities and skills to one outcome: the effective treatment of each individual patient. Mentioned earlier are some of the differences and similarities between management in the private and public sectors. Whatever these differences may be, the ability to break down the various elements of the business or activity and to concentrate upon the key points of each is paramount.

Size and nature of hospital

Questions frequently raised are where are managers for private sector hospitals going to come from, what skills do they require, and indeed what should be the management structure of such hospitals. One of the first papers to look at some of these questions was published in the *Health and Social Services Journal* as a Centre Eight section (Brooks 1985). Some aspects have developed since then and therefore areas of current or common discussion are touched on here.

The starting point clearly has to be the size and nature of the hospital. It does not make economic or practical sense to have a general manager, a director of nursing or matron, and other departmental heads in a hospital that has thirty beds. In setting up any new hospital and even in the larger hospitals, there is a very strong temptation to appoint a manager for every service. The only necessity is the registration require-ment for private hospitals to have a qualified nurse or medical practitioner as the person registered in charge of the unit. When comparing independent hospitals with NHS units there are additional functions, particularly marketing and the extent of the financial organisation within the hospital, requiring in the larger hospital the appointment of a general manager.

It is not necessary to have, say, a separate catering manager and a separate executive housekeeper. Economies of scale can always be achieved providing there are the requisite skills within the hospital to provide the quality of service. If the post of a hotel services manager is used as it is increasingly in some hospitals, that person must be trained in at least one of the areas he or she is expected to be responsible for and therefore acts as the professional head of that section.

The management structure needs to be as lean as possible and the management ladder as short as possible. Many studies have indicated the problems of communication that are experienced as the organisational tree becomes more extended. One of the skills of management is direct communication to all members of staff and the layers of managers and supervisors do not aid this particularly when there is a need — as in all hospitals — to emphasise the concentration on quality and efficiency.

Recruitment

What is the most appropriate recruitment source for general managers of hospitals and what skills should be sought? The most common source, particularly as the independent sector has been growing, has tended to be the NHS on the basis that such recruits know about hospitals, doctors and what health care is about. This background has always been the priority in the minds of some organisations, whilst others have deliberately sought business or other skills. The NHS has experimented with general managers moving into the health care field with various degrees of success, whilst in the private sector with its smaller hospitals it has usually been the skills of the person as opposed to their professional background that have been the determinant of success. Overall the security of tenure for the general manager in the independent sector has increased. Some private health care organisations had a reputation for rapid turnover of their hospital managers with the survival rate being only slightly longer that the life expectancy of an infantry officer in the First World War. As the number of private hospitals has expanded, turnover has decreased as companies have become better at selecting, training and developing such staff.

Whatever the background of a general manager being appointed for the first time to an independent hospital, there is the strong likelihood that they will not have a first hand knowledge of at least some aspects of the work. It may be business finance, marketing or clinical care. Whilst personally I have a slight preference for those who have had some experience of hospitals, in that the ability to relate to consultants and others in their own professional language can often take longer to acquire than some other skills, I am mainly looking for individuals who have high levels of people skills and creativity coupled with common sense. There has to be certain level of personal maturity to allow the rapid absorption of the other skills required. However if there is the strong ability to relate to one's work colleagues, that learning process becomes much easier and considerably faster.

Given the complex nature of hospitals, teamwork and leadership have to be present. It is the general manager's role to ensure that these occur. Special attention needs to be paid to building the teams of professionals who have discrete areas of responsibility so that the working interface between departments is effective.

Another way of looking at the skills required is to consider the 'character' of the general manager. Because private hospitals are 'businesses' — for either profit or surplus — successful hospitals are run by people who can perhaps be categorised as 'hunters'. Such people are required in hospitals that are developing their market-place. There has to be a high energy input into building the reputation and the workload of the hospital with the ability to recognise when services or elements of workload are about to change. That energy must then be concentrated on looking for solutions, alternatives and new ways of marketing the hospital services to the community.

The skill of the hunter needs to be compared with that of the 'farmer'. These latter skills are best suited when a hospital has reached a mature state in its overall development and it is necessary to achieve the best from the existing facilities. Farmers look after the day-to-day business of the hospital. Hunters soon become disillusioned and move when a market has reached maturity - they are looking for other achievements. Therefore, depending upon the stage of development of a hospital from early growth to maturity and possible decline, it may be a farmer or hunter who is the senior manager or chief executive. In general, all managers will have predominance of either 'hunting' or 'farming' in their characters. The excellent manager is one who has been able to develop both areas to the level required for the success of his own particular business and has been able to pull a team around him that complements his own skills and inclinations. There is nothing more frustrating for the visionary than to have to concentrate upon the minutiae of day-to-day work and there must be someone within the management team who is capable of doing that. The hospital whose managers are all hunters will be very successful — for a time — but after a while the cost efficiency will start to slip and other operational problems will become evident including destructive conflict between managers. The hospital that is full of farmers again may be successful for a period of time, but it will become less so as the environment around it changes, requiring the hospital to forecast these changes and to position itself accordingly.

The future hospital managers will be those who can combine an energy, dynamism, creativity and charisma with a practical and persistent approach to the job.

Management principles

Many writers use many different words to describe management, its skills, techniques and tools. The skills necessary for success in the independent sector can be broadly summarised under the headings of general management, marketing, financial and the application of an appropriate amount of clinical understanding. Some necessary attributes in a successful manager are: the ability to communicate, motivate and lead; to have the courage of one's convictions and to delegate; to have a split focus for attention to detail and strategic thinking and achieve a proper balance between the two; to have diplomacy and tact; to be honest and ethical with staff and in the business; to have creativity both in operational efficiency and in longer term planning; to be flexible to changing circumstances but consistent with people and principles. In addition there is the appropriate technical knowledge of one's specific profession or speciality.

Such paragons may be hard to find, but the mix of these skills necessary will depend upon the post itself, the skill mix of other managers, and the internal and external needs of the hospital. For example, a hospital with a declining market share or untapped market opportunities will require a higher level of marketing skills; while people skills may have to be the dominant issue for a manager taking over an unsuccessful hospital with a morale problem.

There are two particular tools of management which I would commend to any manager: outcome thinking and participative management.

Outcome thinking

Outcome thinking is not to be confused with management by objectives. It should also not be regarded as one of the methods of management that go through vogues of acceptability. A hospital's mission must be defined and established, goals and priorities must be set and standards maintained. Because no manager can totally control his environment flexibility of approach and even compromises have to be made. It was only those that Peter Drucker describes as 'misleaders — the Stalins, Hitlers and Maos' who are deluded that compromise is not necessary. But before it is accepted, the manager must have 'thought through what is right and desirable' (Drucker, 1988).

There are many ways of establishing outcomes, particularly when it appears no choices or too many choices are available. The elements of a well-formed outcome are illustrated in Table 2.1.

In using outcome thinking it is necessary to use words with as precise a meaning as possible, and for positive terms to be used. It is a useful tool in achieving a match with the outcomes of others. The technique was developed by Richard Bandler and John Grinder and also expanded by Genie Laborde (1984). It needs practice to obtain the best value.

Participative management

One of the most successful ways of managing is by motivation and one aspect of this is participative management. Whilst the manager sets the goals and the priorities and maintains the standards, he has to be a leader of people. Peter Drucker (1988) wrote 'An effective leader knows that the ultimate task of leadership is to create human energies and human vision.' Examples quoted by Peters and Waterman (1982) and Peters

Table 2.1 Outcomes

Elements	Questions to ask
1 A positive statement of what you want	What do I want? What do I want instead?
2 Evidence	How will I know when I get it? What will I see and hear?
3 Control	What do I do? Is it in my control?
4 Resources	What resources do I have? What new resources can I get? How are they used specifically?
5 Ecology	How will getting this outcome affect everything else? Is it worth it?
6 Action	What is my first step?

and Austin (1985) are paramount in their books indicating that the more people are involved in their own destinies, the greater satisfaction exists and the greater success results. 'Perhaps the most important thing for management is that participation is a long run performance strategy. It is not a panacea nor should it be seen as a stop-gap measure.' (Davis 1981).

The senior manager of a hospital may be committed to participative management, but if it is an alien concept within a hospital it will fall or succeed upon the attitude of departmental or middle managers even though staff may desire it intensely. Alternatively some employees simply want to be left alone to do their job and may be frightened or suspicious of the whole idea.

It therefore must be recognised that there are times when to use and when not to use the technique.

It can be used:

- when changes need to be implemented
- when consensus is needed — when acceptance of the solution is as important as the solution itself
- when better information is needed for making decisions
- when help is needed in identifying the problem
- when help is needed in assessing the group's potential for making a contribution

It should not be used:

• when there is insufficient time for participation
• when the costs of participation exceed the value of the expected results
• when the subject is not relevant to the people asked to participate
• when the people asked to participate are unable to communicate
• when people feel threatened by participating

The process has to be handled carefully and consistently to obtain its full value. It needs to become part of the culture of the hospital. There are many different management styles that can apply and a manager can move from telling someone how a task must be done through to convincing them or selling the task, to allowing participation and ultimately to total delegation. Depending upon the issue to be dealt with and upon the people involved, the manager may swing backwards and forwards between styles. This is situational leadership as developed by Paul Hersey and Ken Blanchard (1982).

Whilst it takes a mature manager to have the courage to delegate and this does necessitate having set an appropriate structure for both the manager and the staff to work within, that maturity of judgment is also needed to recognise in what style the management action should occur. It has often been seen within organisations where immature managers have been told that they must delegate more, and they have done it without allocating the appropriate authority with the responsibility. This on its own is a recipe for a disaster. It is like telling the marketing manager to arrange the marketing strategies and tactics for the hospital and then the hospital director insisting upon doing everything himself, which is both a physical and practical impossibility. Young or immature managers also rely too much on the telling, although this style is appropriate for certain circumstances. When I was commissioning a hospital, pulling together a management team of new managers some of whom had not worked in health care before, there were a number of areas where managers were told what they had to do. In their own particular professional spheres, however, delegation occurred in that the desired outcomes of quality and quantity of services were agreed, and the means by which they were then achieved was that manager's responsibility and each had the authority to carry it out without reference except on the agreed measures.

It is important to note the difference between participation and delegation. Participation obviously means the involvement of people in the management exercise but it also means the final decision rests with the manager. They will have input into the consideration of issues but the final decision rests elsewhere. I refer later to an example where staff of the hospital were involved very much in the design and functional content of an extension to my hospital. That was participative management in that the final decisions rested with myself and my senior managers.

Many hospitals have run specific programmes to develop the management skills at various levels within the organisation and to encourage the participation of managers, supervisors and of staff. One of AMI Healthcare's courses has the title of IER — Involvement, Excellence, Results — which has been a long-running management programme of five years. The intention is that all managers and supervisors should go through this course. It is action oriented which forces people to collaborate and make them think about their styles of management, and it seeks to ingrain some of the easy lessons for management so that they can be applied realistically to the job on a day-to-day basis. The results have been tremendous.

Another useful training tool to develop maturity of decision making and situational leadership has been the involvement of outdoor exercises. In the main, AMI Healthcare has used the Outward Bound organisation. Providing the programmes are properly designed and not just an excuse for a 'bit of fun', worthwhile results have been obtained. The greatest success has been obtained by multi-disciplinary groups and a number of our hospitals have now included supervisory and departmental staff. Whilst there is apprehension from some staff about being involved in physical exercise, and undertaking activities they may never have done before, the environment is designed to be low-risk with individuals maintaining full control over the extent of their own physical involvement. Almost without exception staff enjoy these courses and many lessons have been learnt by both individuals and teams that have been put into practice.

If participation of staff has not been exercised in a particular organisation there are a number of ways of starting the exercise. The following list does not claim to exhaustive but it can be used selectively and expanded upon:-

• Start small with local issues.

• Neither promise nor expect too much.

• Allow people to define for themselves the issues they want to discuss.

• Involve people whose power is at stake.

• Provide education on both the skills of participation, decision making, and the issues that it is decided to pursue initially.

• Maintain leadership by being explicit about the parameters on decisions so that people know how far they can and cannot go.

• Make sure minority views are heard and be wary of group pressure. It is still the manager's right to manage and, as staff become more used to the concept, the danger of group pressure becomes much less in that there is mutual respect for opinion and position.

• Keep time-scales realistic but finite.

• Provide rewards and feedback and tangible signs that the participation mattered and had results.

Built into this whole process should be the ability to think not so much in problems or issues but in outcomes as touched upon earlier. Participative management works, as long as it is worked at hard and consistently.

Management skills

This chapter started off with the statement that management is the application of common sense. One of the *Shorter Oxford English Dictionary* definitions (from 1579) of management is the 'control of courses of affairs by one's own actions.' Whilst the manager works with people to achieve the outcomes, management nevertheless is a personal matter.

The development of common sense starts in infancy and we eventually learn that fire burns or that it hurts to jump off a cliff. Finally we move up the learning ladder from being unconsciously incompetent to being unconsciously competent.

The first general management skill that must develop is a commitment to quality.

Emphasis on quality

In his book *Zen and the Art of Motor Cycle Maintenance*, Robert Pirsig defines quality as 'peace of mind'. Discussion rages in health care on how to define and measure quality.

Peter Drucker wrote in *Adventures of a Bystander* 'Whenever *anything* is being accomplished it is being done, I have learned, by a monomaniac with a mission'. The manager must become the 'monomaniac with a mission' of quality who ensures that his personal zeal for quality is constantly communicated to all staff, users and customers. 'Mission statements' have been mocked in recent years as corny. Used properly however, in staff handbooks, induction days and elsewhere, they can become an effective bench-mark of commitment.

The manager needs to be able to generate a situation which encourages:

* *A concentration upon what the hospital does well*
  Over-diversification usually means that there is insufficient workload to maintain appropriate levels of expertise amongst staff or justify investment in some equipment. Concentrate resources where a high level of skill is possible.

* *The development of skills and resources that achieve success*
  For those areas where the appropriate skills are not available in-house they must be obtained from outside to ensure that each piece of the jigsaw that makes up an efficient hospital is there. Market research and some training facilities, for example, need to be obtained from external specialists.

* *Constant self-criticism*
  An attitude of mind needs to exist amongst all staff that no matter how good something may be today, it can always be better tomorrow. Equally, what is good today may no longer be good tomorrow because circumstances, patients or needs have changed. This requires observation of everything that is going on and seeking feedback from the doctors and patients as to how they are finding things. This must be part of the

culture of the hospital to ensure that staff, as they join the hospital, accept it and work to it.

It will be necessary to overcome the defensive reaction of 'Why change what is working well?' and certainly, change for the sake of change is not appropriate. If however it can be tied in to the general attitude of constantly seeking improvement, the negative aspects of change can be avoided. In fact change can be made into a challenge for everyone within the organisation and the use of working parties, quality circles and suggestion schemes offers but a few of the numerous ways of generating this ongoing interest and commitment.

- *The desire to be the best*
  There have been interminable debates in the health care system over how one measures quality: what are the inputs, what are the outputs and the more subjective issues of judgment of quality. The same difficulty applies to 'what is best?' There is no one definition and in some respects it doesn't matter what the definitions are as long as they are driving the hospital and its people towards success with all that implies for quality and efficiency. Being hypercritical of one's own and other's performance is necessary but has to be handled with care to avoid demotivation. Weaknesses or failures need to be balanced against strengths or successes.

- *An economy of effort*
  This means more than just cost efficiency and using the minimum resource to ensure success. Good time management is a small part of it.

One of the easiest ways of putting across issues of quality to new staff, is to use the phrase 'moments of truth' coined by Jan Carlzon, president of Scandinavian Airlines. Every contact however fleeting with a customer, actual or potential, allows them to make a judgment about an organisation and its efficiency. It is a 'moment of truth'. It also requires something more than a cold clinical approach to efficiency and must demonstrate a genuine warmth for people and their feelings.

Having quality assumes knowing when it exists. The requirement therefore is for constant measurement against preset and regularly revised standards. Means of determining the subjective areas of quality can be, for example, patient questionnaires, use of formal and informal interviews with patient and doctors, the activities of patient liaison officers, quality circles, task forces, market research techniques and quality assurance programmes. One of the most important ways of assessing the quality of a hospital is just by walking about. The managers need to be both highly visible and the catalysts for informed communication with staff, patients and doctors. Tom Peters and others have written too persuasively about 'MBWA' (management by walking about) for it to need further expansion here.

If all these things and more are happening within the hospital, quality can hopefully be 'peace of mind'.

Communication skills

The value of participative management was outlined earlier. The ability to achieve a free flow of communication across a hospital is essential for high quality, motivated staff and satisfied patients.

Two and a half thousand years ago Sun Tzu wrote a book called *The Art of War*. This is still obligatory reading in the Soviet political military hierarchy and was the source of all Mao Tse Tung's strategic and tactical doctrine. It is increasingly being used as a management handbook because whilst dealing with the art of war many of the messages are equally applicable to marketing and management today. In about 100 BC one of Sun Tzu's chroniclers outlined a situation where Sun Tzu in making a point to Ho Lu, king of Wu, drilled on the parade ground 180 ladies from the palace. The ladies did not follow the instructions given and after two attempts Sun Tzu said 'If words of command are not clear and distinct, if orders are not thoroughly understood, the general is to blame. But if his orders are *clear* and the soldiers nevertheless disobey, then it is the fault of their officers.' He then ordered the leaders of the two companies to be beheaded (Sun Tzu, 1981).

Such Draconian measures are not necessary today! But the story serves to illustrate the need to ensure that communication reaches all the way down the line — and back up again. The important point for the manager is to use *all* means of communication effectively and efficiently and to ensure as far as possible that there is consistency of information passing along those lines. It is necessary to establish the means by which information comes back to the manager and that those who sent it can see it as being received, understood, and acted upon. If it is not acted upon, the reason must be communicated back to them.

Lines of informal communication and gossip within hospitals are prolific. The situation has to be accepted — and managed — to ensure that wrong messages which could lead to loss of motivation and a fall in standards and even staff leaving, are avoided. Positive messages can also be passed very effectively through these lines. Again this calls for high visibility from the senior managers within the hospital and organisation. It emphasises the need to maximise the involvement of all members of staff in the many aspects of hospital life, planning and its future. It includes that attention to detail; it leads to that combined effort towards excellence.

If you ask the right questions of your staff you will sometimes be surprised at the answers you receive. When starting to plan one of the major extensions to my former hospital in Manchester, I decided to seek the views of the hospital staff as to its siting, layout, content, etc. They would, after all, be working in the completed building. It has long been accepted, particularly in the NHS, that you cannot plan a building by committee. However at a special meeting, the staff were given certain information as to the overall site and design constraints imposed by the local planning committee and an outline of what the building needed to contain. They were asked to consider what impact the new wing with its extra patients, staff and demand on services would have on the rest of the hospital, how the extension would best fit onto the site, and what should be the functional relationship of rooms and services. By working in small groups the results were outstanding with remarkable consistency of view, and it was possible to incorporate many of the suggestions into the design. Over one-third of the hospital staff took part in that exercise and the degree of ownership felt towards the extension whilst it was being built and subsequently operated was tremendous. The value of the exercise also went beyond the original outcomes in that the same means were subsequently used to obtain agreement on a no smoking policy within the hospital which was then implemented without any problems.

Whilst these two small examples dealt with specific issues, communication within the hospital obviously has to occur on an ongoing basis. The information coming from the top has to be honest, accurate and consistent coupled with an open-door policy and a desire to receive feedback and to act upon it.

Communication with one's customers, whether patient, consultant, employer or visitor, is equally important and there are different ways of approaching each customer that are specific to his own particular needs. In AMI Healthcare's internal quality assurance programmes, emphasis is laid upon the ability of staff to communicate with one another which ensures quality and a teamwork approach in the view of patients. One of the ill-informed criticisms of the private sector used to be that the hospitals were staffed by part-timers or agency staff. That is clearly not so, but the nurses do have to face the fact that patients on the whole are in single- or two-bedded rooms as opposed to the old Nightingale wards or open bays of the NHS. Therefore it is incumbent upon our nurses to pay more attention to individual contact and communication than perhaps is actually necessary in an open ward. Various studies carried out by AMI Healthcare have demonstrated how patient perceptions can change from simply seeing a nurse even though no direct communication may have occurred. As with a manager, visibility coupled with accessibility are essential aids to effective communication.

Building work in hospitals always causes problems of noise and therefore potential patient dissatisfaction. Even this situation can be managed as the AMI Alexandra Hospital in Manchester showed with its extensions. This was done by involving the patients in the scheme and its progress even before they were admitted to hospital. Despite the major physical disruption to the site, the level of problem experienced was in terms of communication and also of physical screening. One outcome was that some patients requested a room with a view of the building work.

Independent hospitals need to market their services so that consultants, general practitioners, employers, potential patients are aware of what is available. A consistency of message is essential. Whatever the means of that communication, whether personal visits, major presentations, use of written material, market research or other means, the culture or ethos of the hospital must be demonstrated by the professionalism, warmth and interest of the people concerned. Communication between hospital staff serves to make the communication and service to the hospital's customers more effective. It is occasionally necessary to remember that those issues that may be important to staff at a given time will not necessarily be the priorities of a doctor or of a patient just admitted. A balance of priorities has to be maintained.

Dual focus

One of the major issues facing health care over the next decade will be shortages in manpower. Seven out of ten people in the workforce of the year 2000 are already working. By the same time the NHS will need to employ 40 per cent of all female school leavers with 5 good GCSEs. Add the fact that most employers tend to recruit from the 18-25 age group, and further problems for the future are only too clear. Appropriate recruitment, retention and development of staff are going to require strategic creativity and the motivation of staff on a day-to-day basis. It is but one example of how managers need to demonstrate an aptitude for another skill of long term planning.

There can be no dispute that the ability to plan properly for the future is a prerequisite for business success. There can equally be no denying that managers must pay attention to detail of the operational aspects of their hospital. Some managers have the ability to concentrate on one but not both areas. If this is so, efforts should be made to develop this dual focus. If the chief executive officer or hospital director, as he must, is concerned about the quality of service that is provided, he must demonstrate his interest in that attention to detail at all levels throughout his organisation. How this is done will be a matter of personal preference but, as usual, actions are more effective than words. For example, it irritates me if when I go into a shop, a restaurant or a hospital I see remnants of Christmas decorations, so there was a good-natured competition between myself and the housekeeping staff in the Alexandra after the twelfth day of Christmas to see whether any sellotape or other remnants had been left on the ceilings, tops of cupboards or whatever. The investment of my time was absolutely minimal but the message was clear and the principle was carried on by my staff throughout the year. This is just an example of an extremely minor item but it possibly serves to demonstrate an attitude of mind to detail to achieve the essential operational efficiency of a hospital.

The perception of the customer is the important thing. Peters and Austin (1985) outline many examples of the way in which attention to detail or lack of it influenced customer perception. One example from the airline industry quoted there, was that if the flip-down trays had coffee stains on them the likelihood was that equal lack of attention had been paid to the maintenance of the engines. If a patient's room has not been cleaned properly what is the likelihood that the same situation applies in the operating theatres? Or if a nurse does not have her hair tidily in place, is she going to be equally careless about her hands-on care of the patient?

Sir William Osler once wrote ' The best preparation for tomorrow is to do today's work superbly well'. When a hospital is able to generate a culture of quality and operates in a location where there are sufficient people who want to and are able to buy that service, the likelihood of success is extremely strong. However in John Harvey-Jones's words, 'today's success is all too often tomorrow's failure. This can happen when the way we do things around here .... rests on the assumption that what has worked well in the past may work well in the future.' (1988).

Health care is in a particularly fast changing environment in the late 1980s and a manager needs to take account of technological trends and more particularly, of what is happening in his general market-place. The 1989 Government White Paper is intended to change dramatically the way in which patients' care is organised and funded. The proposals in that White Paper present both opportunities and threats to the private sector. An organisation's ability to recognise these and act upon them is important. There is a changing relationship between the hospital providers and the third party payers. Traditional health insurance is not meeting totally the needs of a growing proportion of the insured population, and the provident associations together with the commercial insurance companies are looking at their own futures. Coupled with this there will be the likely growth of companies like Medisure and Remedi who are the interface between the purchaser of private health-care facilities and the providers themselves with much greater attention being paid to the management of such costs. The pattern of ownership within the private health-care sector is also changing and therefore the activities of one's competition have increasing importance. Of a more fundamental nature there will be, as mentioned earlier, the increasing shortage of skills over the next few years.

With the day-to-day pressures of running a hospital, and particularly one in an organisation or situation where short term budget achievement is a high priority, the ability to look forward is quickly driven out by Gresham's law of day-to-day pressures preventing long term planning. A balance must be struck and that is why the ability of a manager to have a dual focus between day-to-day detail and long term planning is essential.

Marketing issues

In the opinion of one health authority chairman 'Concepts such as marketing, advertising and public relations might seem to be part of an alien culture and smack of something not quite savoury.' (Higgins, 1988).

Indeed marketing is perhaps the one area that managers, particularly those from the NHS, entering the independent health care sector are most apprehensive about. There are concerns on the part of some people that marketing is not appropriate to the provision of health care, but more positively these days there is an increasing recognition in all walks of life that effective marketing is an essential activity in developing a business or service. It is appropriate that hospitals and health care organisations should employ people with professional marketing skills. However the general manager is expected to have an understanding of the subject and has an important role to play in the overall marketing activities of the unit or business. Marketing is an essential and integral part of management.

At hospital level *every* member of the staff no matter what his or her job within the hospital, has a marketing role. It may be in relation to patients or visitors they meet within the hospital; it may be how they portray the hospitals to their friends and contacts outside by what they say; how they behave can influence whether others wish to come and work at or be treated in the hospital.

To understand this one has to understand what marketing actually is. Rather like management there are many definitions and the principle of marketing has been misunderstood and under-utilised by many in the health care field. It tends to be defined in terms of its most visible aspects, i.e. sales, promotion, public relations and advertising. A much broader and better definition is that: 'Marketing is the effective identification and management of exchange relationships.' (AMI Healthcare, 1988).

The 'exchange' is the central concept underlying marketing and the central activity of the business, in other words both parties — the vendor and the buyer, or the hospital and the patient or other customer — must be satisfied with the outcome. The patient must be satisfied with the treatment and care received whilst in the hospital and that value for money has occurred. The hospital must be satisfied that it has firstly provided the level of care and facilities that is appropriate to the level of quality it seeks to maintain; secondly the whole episode has been carried out in a cost-efficient manner; and thirdly it has been paid for its services. Thus marketing is a managerial process and not just something which 'the marketing people' do nor is it restricted solely to advertising.

To achieve that exchange relationship the marketing has to be identified and managed. The activities involved in this are: analysis; planning; implementation; and control.

Market areas, such as acute care, psychiatry, long-stay care are selected and whilst the private health-care sector can clearly do this and NHS cannot, the lack of freedom to select a market-place in detail is not particularly important as long as the following steps are taken. The market's needs are researched and the organisation's offerings are designed to meet these needs rather than in the terms of the seller's needs or wants. Price, the means of promotion and the means of delivery of the service or product are also an integral part.

Managers must ensure that their organisation's marketing is an integral part of its overall activities. Philip Kotler, a renowned authority on the subject, once observed that market orientated organisations shared five common characteristics and these serve as a useful summary of what good marketing requires (Kotler and Clarke, 1987):

• A customer philosophy.

• An ingrained marketing organisation.

• Adequate market information systems.

• A strategic orientation.

• Operational efficiency.

The application of these is expanded upon by Paul McDevitt (1987) who emphasises once again that a strategic view must be taken and the active role that must be taken by the chief executive officer or hospital director.

In the past, parts of the private sector have tended to bleat about unfair competition from the NHS with heavily subsidised pay beds, and the bias in the distribution of waiting list initiatives moneys since medical fees and overheads did not need to be considered by the NHS.

The independent sector exists because of choice — by users and providers. It does not matter if one part of the market-place operates under different rules. It is the opportunity for the independent manager to create something different. The ability to think strategically about the market-place is essential otherwise the opportunities — and threats — arising from the 1989 White Paper will be lost.

The important issues are to ensure the hospital is always looking to its market-places, the levels of satisfaction and taking the longer term view that respectively optimises and combats the opportunities and threats that may occur. In addition 'exchange relationships' need to multiply.

Financial issues

The basic issue that many people come across for the first time when entering the independent sector is the need for the hospital to earn money as well as controlling expenditure. It perhaps affects nurses and departmental staff the most when they have to keep records of what is used on behalf of each patient or even have to ask for money. In my experience it takes many staff up to six months to learn to cope with this. Some cannot and sadly leave.

Hospital managers and departmental managers have to learn how to use and control budgets. Management ratios are a useful tool in this respect and each manager will be able to develop those which best suit his own purposes. There is often a temptation to initiate too many control systems with too many pieces of paper. Avoid it — keep things as simple as possible within the bounds of good accounting and audit practice.

One part of the financial equation is worth highlighting: pricing. The issue of pricing has to be learnt. In the past it was relatively easy in that perhaps the hospital charged at or below what insurance companies were willing to reimburse. Those days are gone for many hospitals with there being a greater mismatch between reimbursement and charge. It is not appropriate to take the basic cost of an item or service and add a margin for overheads, and maybe profit. Other factors in addition to cost have to be taken into account such as the market position of the hospital - high value or low cost, comparison with competitors, understanding what drives demand for each particular service as well as the rate and speed of return required. Market research can often aid the introduction of realistic pricing levels. Once again the pervasive nature of marketing is apparent.

One final point on financial matters relates to cost efficiency. Whilst recognising that every action has a cost, it is equally important that manager and staff do not have a mind-set that cost saving is always the order of the day — unless it has to be of course. But cost efficiency, or cost management, must occur with proper cost-control systems, particularly on labour, supplies and fees, as well as recognising that capital investment on equipment such as energy-saving devices can also achieve the same ends. Robert Heller in his book *The New Naked Manager* spelt out his rules of management: his tenth rule was that the easiest way of making money was to stop losing it. Haemorrhaging of money can be equally fatal!

Clinical understanding

An area of knowledge mentioned earlier which can affect the recruitment source of a general manager is the level of awareness of health care in general and clinical matters in particular.

Unless the professional background of a general manager is indeed clinical he can never seek to match the level of knowledge of his professional clinical staff and the doctors using the hospital. What is more important is that the manager is capable of showing an understanding of the needs of clinicians, an awareness of the type of work they do, the major service requirements of their specialty, and some of the complications, problems and issues they face. It is perhaps questionable whether this knowledge is needed right from the very beginning provided that within the management structure there is someone at a senior level, for example a director of nursing, who can provide the necessary clinical guidance to the general manager. The role of a medical advisory committee is also critical in this respect.

There is a higher value on being a good listener with the ability to organise, to plan, to communicate and to ensure an efficient operation overall.

Most certainly the general manager is going to have to keep himself up to date with the technological and clinical changes that are likely to occur. Only in this way can the strategic future of the hospital be considered seriously. The pace of change is increasing and the manager needs to recognise the value of developments in information technology, applied medicine and the new technologies of, for example, magnetic resonance imaging, SPECT (single photon emission computed tomography), and the potential value of PET (positron emission tomography). There are also the changes in treatment technologies such as lithotripsy, the use of medical lasers and genetic engineering.

If a manager is maintaining the necessary degree of contact with his medical staff, an appropriate knowledge and understanding can soon be acquired simply by that contact and selected intelligent reading and attendance at appropriate lectures. For example, the Institute of Health Services Management ran in 1989 a very successful series of lectures on 'Medicine for Managers'.

Outsiders have tended on occasions to take the view that there is not much difference between running hotels and hospitals and the private sector is currently seeing growing interest from leisure management groups in moving into health care. One of the worst criticisms a private hospital can receive is for a private patient to say ' You're a good hotel but a poor hospital.' The way of combating this is by emphasising clinical and non-clinical standards and working very closely with the doctors using the hospital.

Doctors have become more used to general managers within the NHS who have not had previous health care experience. Whilst some of these acquaintances have proved to be unhappy for both parties, there have been many success stories, proving that good management skills can work in any environment. The private sector is no exception to this.

Honesty in management

I have outlined some of the areas of skill successful managers in health care — and elsewhere — need to develop. There is an attitude of mind that cannot be developed but must be inherent in all of us and that is the honest and ethical nature of our personal and business behaviour.

In the past many external commentators have questioned the morality of the existence of the private sector and whether it can justify allowing people to jump queues simply by virtue of their wealth. My point is not to argue the social equity model of our society but simply to emphasise once again a very self-evident issue. Namely, that the reputation and the success of a hospital and organisation come about because of its ethics and morality as well as its quality. Rumours have long abounded in medicine about payments being made for the referral of patients, of letters being given to overseas patients to enable them to circumnavigate their country's currency regulations, and of consultants using NHS equipment without permission in private hospitals.

The external business ethics of any hospital and organisation have to be impeccable. Equally impeccable has to be the relationship between the manager and his staff. Hidden pressures on staff in the hope that they will leave, ducking the issue when unpleasant questions are asked, promising to do something it is not intended to carry out, are all unacceptable practices for a manager. If a hospital has problems, sharing them with the staff can often bring surprising results. Many of the staff will rally round, recognising they are being fairly treated and responding accordingly. Those that cannot cope with the situation are likely to either leave or be subject to peer pressure and improve their performance. However it is no use for a manager who has a reputation for not being straight with his staff to suddenly come to them and say that he wishes to share a problem. Ulterior motives will be suspected. In the case of unsatisfactory performance by a member of staff, counselling and constructive attempts to change the situation may be painful at the time, but will earn the manager respect from other staff even if dismissal of an individual is the end result. They will appreciate being dealt with fairly.

If a manager can deal with the difficult situations honestly and fairly, they will in fact — at least internally — become less and less, and more time can be spent upon the opportunities for growth and development.

Conclusion

With two minor exceptions, I have not touched upon the 'science' of management and described market research and planning techniques, labour management systems etc. but concentrated rather upon 'the art of management'. Many books have been written about both aspects of management and I simply offer my personal and deliberately simplistic view of management.

There is nothing profound, or new in what I have described, but the application of common sense, working with our people, keeping it simple and most important having that overriding commitment to quality is 'management'. Health care, because it is about people at their most vulnerable, must have first class management in both the independent and public sectors.

Winning will come from quality, service, incredible responsiveness, constant adaptation, extraordinary commitment from large numbers of passionate champions. In other words, winning is one hundred per cent from people. Leadership of people is anything but a bloodless business and above all depends upon commitment, care, energy, love of the product and care for what you are doing. (Peters, *The world turned upside down* (Thames TV video)).

Further reading

Listed below are some of the books I have enjoyed or found useful in my practice of management. Some can be skimmed, others need a more studied approach. I hope some of them will be of use.

Aaron HJ, Schwartz WB 1984 *The painful prescription*. Brookings Institution

Albrecht K, Zenke R 1985 *Service America*. Dow Jones Irwin

Bennis W, Nanus B 1985 *Leaders*. Harper & Row

Bonama TV 1985 *The marketing edge*. Macmillan

Carzon J 1987 *Moment of truth*. Ballinger Publishing

de Bono E 1987 *Letters to thinkers*. Harrap

Deal TE, Kennedy AA 1982 *Corporate cultures*. Addison Wesley

Freemantle D 1985 *Super boss*. Gower

Goldsmith W, Clutterbuck D 1984 *The winning streak*. Weidenfeld & Nicolson

Goldsmith W, Clutterbuck D 1985 *The winning streak workout book*. Weidenfeld & Nicolson

Harvey-Jones J 1988 *Making it happen*. Collins

Heller R 1980 *The business of winning*. Guild Publishing

Heller R 1985 *The new naked manager*. Hodder & Stoughton

Heller R 1984 *The super managers*. Sidgwick & Jackson

Hersey P, Blanchard K 1982 *Management of organisational behaviour*. 4th edn. Prentice-Hall

Heskett J L, 1986 *Managing in the service economy*. Harvard Business School Press

Hickman C, Silva MA 1984 *Creating excellence.* George Allen & Unwin
Higgins J 1988 *The business of medicine.* Macmillan Education
Kiam V 1986 *Going for it!* Collins
Koestenbaum P 1987 *The heart of business.* Saybrook Publishing
Laborde GZ 1984 *Influencing with integrity.* Syntony Publishing
Leboeuf M 1986 *How to motivate people.* Sidgwick & Jackson
McCormack MH 1984 *What they don't teach you at Harvard Business School.* Collins
McLachlan G, Maynard A (eds) 1982 *The public/private mix for health.* Nuffield Provincial Hospitals Trust
Peters T 1987 *Thriving on chaos.* Alfred A Knopf
Peters TJ Waterman RH 1982 *In search of excellence.* Harper & Row
Peters TJ, Austin N 1985 *A passion for excellence.* Random House
Ries A, Trout J 1986 *Marketing warfare.* McGraw-Hill
Robbins A 1986 *Unlimited power.* Fawcett Columbine
Sun Tzu, 1981 *The art of war,* edited by J Clavell. Hodder & Stoughton
von Oech R *1983 A whack on the side of the head.* Creative Think

References

AMI Healthcare 1988 *Strategic market management* (Internal document)
Brooks T 1985 Private care *Health & Social Services Journal* Centre Eight Section 21 Nov 1981
Davis PA 1981 Building a workable participative management system *Management Review* Mar.: 39-44
Drucker P 1988 Leadership: more doing than dash. *Wall Street Journal* 6 Jan: 67-70
Harvey-Jones J 1988 *Making it happen.* Collins
Hersey P, Blanchard K 1982 *Management of organizational behaviour.* 4th edn. Prentice-Hall
Higgins J 1988 *The business of medicine.* Macmillan Education
Kotler P, Clarke RN 1987 *Marketing for healthcare organizations.* Prentice-Hall
McDevitt P 1987 Learning by doing: strategic marketing management in hospitals. *Health Care Management Review* **12** (1): 23-30
Sun Tzu 1981 *The art of war,* edited by J Clavell. Hodder & Stoughton

3 Finance
John Rigby Jones

As with any organisation, all elements are crucial, and it is difficult to rank the relative importance of those elements. Certainly, within private health care, finance skills are critical, and the achievement of financial goals essential. This chapter covers the whole field, from issues of capital funding, through to detailed budgeting skills.

Background

The private hospital industry is small and prone to public misconception and political misrepresentation but it can offer real challenges to the open-minded and objective financial executive. Key and often unique aspects to the industry include the high level of fixed operating costs and the slow maturity cycle of a hospital; the critical restrictions imposed by hospital capacity and the requirements for continuous reinvestment; the high proportion and wide range of professional staff employed; the dominance of one major customer; its growth potential, and its disparate nature.

Internally the industry has a wide range of corporate structures. Its major players have included registered charities, both religious and otherwise, subsidiaries of American health care companies, public companies, subsidiaries of leisure or hotel companies, overseas investment companies, and provident associations. Their differing abilities to obtain financial and fiscal advantages have often been insufficiently understood by their competitors. Its external relationships are largely not with corporations but with individuals, both patients and doctors, and provident associations whose financial perspective can be radically different from that of the corporation.

It is an industry at a crossroads. Just as 'Big Bang' was the catalyst whereby financial power in the City of London was concentrated in the hands of a few major players plus some successful niche players but with small and unadventurous players going out of business, so that challenging prospect now faces the private hospital industry. Nevertheless there remains great scope for growth through the development of new services and insurance products to reflect and create new demand.

Revenue

Bed occupancy

Like the hotel industry, the private hospital industry is one where, despite the increasing importance of ancillary revenues, bed occupancy remains critical. This is especially so since operating costs are largely fixed by nature because of both the high capital costs of a hospital investment (as evidenced by the relationship between turnover and investment) and the need to staff a high number of small departments regardless of occupancy on a close to continuous basis.

Measured as patient days (or bed nights) charged, average daily census (often counted at midnight), or as a percentage of available or licensed beds, annual occupancy can rarely exceed 75 per cent because of weekly and monthly fluctuations in admissions. Patients, and more especially doctors, may avoid an admission at weekends or during holiday periods. It can even fluctuate dramatically during a day. The ability to predict likely admission trends and then to control operating costs by maximising flexibility is critical in achieving profitability and competitive advantage.

Unlike the hotel industry no two customers receive exactly the same service; and one cannot rely on repeat business for future success. Additional complications for the hospital are a wider range of services and revenue-earning departments, a much larger number of charges (with up to 500 commonly recognised surgical procedures and 3000 different drugs and medical supplies in stock), and a room rate which includes 24-hour medical monitoring and room service.

It is vital also to appreciate the roles of patient, doctor, and, where appropriate, insurer as customer. The patient is the recipient of the service; the doctor (both general practitioner and consultant) is the main decision maker regarding utilisation and is also the partial provider of that service; and, where the patient is insured, the insurance company is the payer. All must be considered in a hospital's marketing plan and by the financial manager in accumulating meaningful occupancy statistics.

Breakdown of hospital revenue

A hospital invoice for an inpatient will usually include charges for accommodation (usually inclusive of routine nursing and catering), the use of the theatre and paramedical departments, the provision of pharmaceutical and medical supplies, and other hotel-related charges: the last is usually not covered by medical insurance and may require separate billing. A patient will usually receive additional invoices from the surgeon for both surgery and pre- and post-operative consultations and from the anaesthetist for anaesthesia during surgery. There will usually be no direct financial relationship between a consultant surgeon and a hospital.

Excluding Central London, where an albeit reduced overseas market remains important, approximately 80 per cent of inpatients admitted to private hospitals are covered by private health insurance. Of this approximately 60 per cent are covered by the British United Provident Association (BUPA), followed by Private Patients' Plan (PPP) and a number of smaller insurers including Western Provident Association (WPA) and Bristol Contributory Welfare Association(BCWA). With such a high dependence on one group of customers and so dominant a market-leader within that group it is essential both to maintain good relations and to understand fully the varying services covered by their products.

Role of the insurer

Levels of insured medical cover may be restricted, often excluding pre-existing medical conditions and limiting the amount claimable annually for a particular benefit. Again cover is usually restricted to acute medical or surgical conditions with certain conditions totally excluded of which the patient, through lack of advice or understanding, may be ignorant. These typically include possibly open-ended and unsuccessful treatments of great expense, such as organ transplantation, dialysis, and AIDS, and treatments that are either not deemed acute or which may be avoided at the insuree's choice, such as alcohol, drug, or psychiatric therapy, routine dentistry, and childbirth where surgical intervention is not required. A justification can be made for these limitations as they will have been excluded from the actuarial calculation of premium levels — in the United States they are usually at least partially covered and premiums are correspondingly many times higher — but may cause problems for the hospital: in this and many other respects the insurer is shielded from his customer by the hospital. Through patient ignorance and insurer reticence a hospital will often be unable to confirm limitations to a patient's cover prior to treatment, and thereby establish the eventual payer for its services and indeed the price if the insurers have negotiated discounted prices.

The insurers have historically offered a range of products and premiums which were linked to NHS private pay-bed rates and had a high degree of regional variation. The increase in multi-banding, whereby hospitals have successfully negotiated to accept more than one range of insured patient without the insurers short-falling reimbursement at the expense of either the patient or the hospital, has reduced such variation. Variations in the price of the premiums and hospital charges increasingly reflects only the perceived quality of a hospital's hotel services — every patient will receive the same standard of medical care — or the skill of a hospital's price negotiation. As a result location, always a prime consideration for a hospital's success, is an increasingly important factor in hospital profitability not least because there are wide regional variations in hospital costs, especially the salaries of both medical and ancillary staff.

Additionally, variations in the cost of premiums are unevenly spread with a large difference between the highest rate and a number of cheaper ones: the market should eventually dictate the need for a more even spread of choice. Nevertheless both hospitals and insurers have gained from the public's inverse view of the normal price/demand relationship. Health care and the price of health care are widely misunderstood: the consumers' assumption to date has been that increased price reflects increased quality. Nobody to date has attempted to classify private hospitals on the basis of quality, however measured, or range of services rather than price.

The advantages of a successful price contract, usually negotiated annually, with an insurer can be great in spite of a frequently perceived loss of independence. It will probably lead to a higher level of reimbursement for insured patients, inclusion in insurance literature, patient reassurance that his bill will be paid and his treatment satisfactory, and improvement in debt collection. A hospital will usually send its bill directly to an insurer together with the relevant claim documentation and will be reimbursed regularly and directly. Without a contract the bill will be sent to the patient who will either be financially inconvenienced if he pays promptly or will wait until he himself is reimbursed.

The cover provided by insurance tends to be split into a number of benefits reimbursable to a hospital; given the market share of the insured patient, a hospital's billing system tends to adopt this split for all patients. The main benefits are accommodation, theatre fees, drugs and dressings, and ancillary services. This method of billing is usually called 'fee for item of service' with drugs and dressings either charged individually or in a number of inclusive packs. Theatre fees themselves are subdivided into five categories of surgical procedure — minor, intermediate, major, major plus, and complex. This subdivision is based more on the complexity of surgery within theatre than the overall time and cost of hospital care. There can be widely different average lengths of a patient's stay for different operations in the same category. Consequently, while this subdivision may provide hospital management with the easiest classification of patient mix, it can be misleading.

Other methods of reimbursement may resolve this problem and at the same time reduce patient and insurer uncertainty about the level of hospital charges: they may also radically alter the financial relationship and transfer insurance risk between insurer and provider. Various types of inclusive charge, whether by day or by admission, are already common and are likely to increase.

Arrangements such as the diagnostic related groupings (DRGs) introduced by the United States government for the reimbursement of state-sponsored patients, whereby each surgical procedure is given its own all-inclusive reimbursement rate per admission, will eventually reach this country. It is already standard practice to offer such 'package' prices, often discounted but subject to limitations in length of stay, to uninsured patients as a means of both reducing patient uncertainty about cost and encouraging high-profit marginal business. These prices are usually well-publicised and market-driven. And, as has happened dramatically in the United States, hospitals become considerably more financially exposed to inadequate cost control.

The present system of a fee for each item of service has allowed hospitals to ensure a mark-up on each component of service, especially in the area of drugs and dressings where costs have run ahead of inflation. Those hospitals that have reviewed or agreed their supplies charges annually in advance will have lost out to those who, usually through computerised stock control, have been able to perform more frequent or even on-line price reviews.

Other revenue statistics

After occupancy the key revenue statistic is unit revenue per patient, either by day or admission. Variations in this figure will correspond to variations in patient mix, either in the complexity of surgery or, where there is differential pricing, in patient classification, or will highlight the efficiency of a hospital's revenue capture systems. Variations will be further highlighted by a breakdown of revenue into its component parts since some charges are linked directly to the number of admissions (such as theatre charges) and others to patient days (such as room charges). But such a breakdown has often been compared to a balloon: when the market squeezes one benefit, charges for other benefits tend to increase to compensate — the balloon always stays the same size. In the same way hospital departments are at the same time separate entities but part of an integrated service.

It is also important to differentiate gross and net revenue. Levels of discounts of up to 25 per cent in the United States have made gross revenue increasingly unrealistic with it being said cynically that gross revenue is what one would like to charge and net revenue what one is allowed to charge. Calculations based on gross revenue may therefore be unrealistic when provided to management.

Pricing

There is a lack of published guidelines as to what a hospital or consultant does and may properly charge, although most hospitals will have some idea of their immediate competitors' charges. The high fixed element within costs and the individuality of each patient and doctor — a review of theatre times and costs to perform the same operation underlines this — makes pricing based on cost difficult, although the 'fee for item of service' method of charging certainly helps to differentiate the cost of components and ensure adequate mark-up on each. Most hospitals will be able to assess which operations produce the most revenue: few will be able to say which are the most profitable. Management may feel it important to be able to undertake all types of surgery regardless of profitability and it is indeed headstrong to hope to encourage a consultant surgeon to undertake one operation in his specialty but not another when he is not subject to the same profit constraints; nevertheless it is better to take that decision in defiance of the facts rather than in the absence of them.

Some prices are certainly based on demand and competition — especially inclusive prices for the uninsured — and such published prices, usually loss-leaders, may attract new patients and, more especially, new consultants who may thereby be encouraged for the sake of convenience to bring other more profitable business. A doctor would naturally prefer to do a full operating session in one hospital rather than two split sessions in different hospitals.

The major advantage of high fixed costs is the high profitability of even low-priced marginal business, especially if that business can be timed to suit the hospital. In some cases the cost of treating an additional patient, where there is spare capacity in staffing, accommodation, and theatre time, may be restricted almost to the cost of supplies, food, and paramedical tests and is thus more easy to price. The dangers of such pricing are, firstly, that marginal business may increasingly become core business, thus radically altering cost analyses: and, secondly, that core business, and especially insurers, may react unfavourably in the same way that full-fare paying train or aeroplane passengers may to cut-price travel. Reconciliation of the two may require setting normally unacceptable constraints on the availability of these prices such as type of room or time of treatment.

Other revenue

Whilst inpatient business has been the historical bedrock of the industry, day-case, outpatient, and other business, including the rental of onsite consulting rooms to consultants, has and will become increasingly important and now probably accounts for up to 25 per cent of revenue and over 80 per cent of customers. The reasons are manifold.

Firstly, improvements in medical technology, surgical technique, post-operative treatment, and even administrative planning continue to reduce the average length of an inpatient stay and in some cases have prevented the need for an overnight stay completely. Secondly, the resultant price reduction has been successfully marketed to a wider patient base. Thirdly, such marketing has given the hospital access to the patient at an earlier stage and has thus won customer and brand awareness and loyalty. Fourthly, it has attached the general practitioner more formally to the hospital as part of the patient referral base and on occasion enabled him to be rewarded when in the past private health care was and was perceived to be largely the domain of the consultant physician or surgeon. Fifthly, increased public awareness of health and health care issues has caused a demand for the type of preventative medicine, not least health screening, that state-of-the-art technology and a private hospital's outpatient facilities can offer.

Lastly, whereas a private hospital needed paramedical departments such as pathology, physiotherapy, and radiology to be seen to provide a comprehensive inpatient service, the necessary investment could only be justified if likely utilisation far exceeded inpatient requirements alone. Thus for many hospitals the development of outpatient workload has been no more than a method of diluting inpatient costs, with the majority of radiology and physiotherapy revenue now coming from outpatient referrals.

Costs

If occupancy is the key factor in ensuring an adequate return on an investment in a private hospital then proper cost management, allied with skillful pricing of marginal business, can minimise losses or maximise profits. Given the long maturity cycle of a hospital, cost management is especially important in the early years of an investment: more than one hospital has suffered from over-optimistic projections of occupancy growth and thus overspent on largely fixed costs which it has been subsequently difficult to prune.

It is essential always to maintain the maximum cost flexibility without reducing quality of service. In the early years this may mean subcontracting services which would be inappropriate in a mature hospital. An in-house pathology service, for example, is expensive to establish in staffing, equipping and stockholding terms: it may be advantageous to subcontract pathology initially. The same may be said with less force for other revenue-earning departments such as radiology, physiotherapy, and pharmacy or indeed overhead departments such as laundry, housekeeping, and catering. There is wide disparity within the industry as to what departments it is appropriate and cost effective to subcontract.

Costs are usually broken down by natural classification and by department, of which there are many, both revenue-earning and overhead, in even the smallest hospital. These would include nursing services (primarily wards, outpatients, and theatre), paramedical services (such as radiology, pathology, physiotherapy, and pharmacy), hotel services (laundry, housekeeping, reception and telephonists, and catering), support services (stores, maintenance and portering) and administration (hospital director, director of nursing, accounting and business office).

The major components of cost by natural classification are salaries, probably accounting for 35 per cent to 50 per cent of revenue, medical and other supplies, probably accounting for 10 per cent to 20 per cent, medical fees (5 per cent), subcontracted services, administrative and hotel overheads, and property and finance costs. The wide variations in the above costs as percentages of revenue depend primarily on occupancy, patient characteristics and the extent to which services have been subcontracted. However most mature hospitals should aim at an operating profit margin before property and finance costs (which may vary considerably according to the financial structure of the group) of at least 30 per cent.

Salaries and staffing costs

The control of staffing costs, the largest cost element, is obviously of paramount importance. Medical and other professional staff can attract high salaries and, with the exception of nursing, they will usually be expected to work in small departments. The appointment of the right calibre of working supervisor is critical: as budget holders, with little and different financial experience obtained from their NHS career, they will probably need a high degree of financial training to ensure their overall departmental financial responsibility including proper revenue capture and cost control systems.

Since occupancy varies dramatically over the short and longer term it is inappropriate to employ full-time or even contracted part-time staff to cover fully the peaks in occupancy and thereby be overstaffed at the time of the troughs. For smaller departments this can largely be overcome by judicious use of overtime working, flexible working hours, and proper holiday planning. For larger departments, primarily ward and theatre nursing, such methods are insufficiently sophisticated.

Proper control in these departments requires: first, as much prior knowledge of projected occupancy as possible — although emergency admissions can upset even the best run department; secondly, a methodology for establishing the staffing levels required for different occupancy and case-mix levels, usually measured in terms of either full-time equivalent (FTE) numbers of staff or hours worked or paid: thirdly, a method of comparing actual and expected staffing levels; and, lastly, an understanding of the most efficient way of accommodating a given occupancy — is the staffing of one full ward more efficient that that of two half-full wards? The established way of providing flexibility in nursing is through the use of bank nurses, non-contracted staff usually provided with uniforms but without fixed working hours. Most often compared to 'supply' teachers, they provide the short-term flexibility that part-time staff cannot. Part-time staff, unless the timing of their contracted hours is at the hospital's discretion, are only a solution for and have usually been appointed in anticipation of a longer-term occupancy growth where the appointment of full-time staff cannot be justified.

Short-term occupancy shortages can also be covered by the use of overtime or agency nurses but may be less cost-effective. A rough guideline may be to staff on a full-time basis up to 75 per cent to 80 per cent of expected annual occupancy with the balance being covered by bank staff. A lower full-time complement causes problems in getting the right number of bank staff when required, a lack of continuity and understanding of the hospital's nursing practices and other anomalies such as uniforms, staff loyalty and commitment. A higher complement will lead to overstaffing at periods of low occupancy.

It is equally important to minimise those peaks and troughs in occupancy. On a short-term or weekly basis the administrator with spare theatre capacity may avoid bottlenecks by better theatre planning and incentives for using the theatre at off-peak times. On a longer term basis, use of marginal prices at off-peak times to fill empty but fully-nursed beds can be successful. Proper theatre planning should also ensure the correct timing of day-case patients, where there is an obvious deadline, if the patient is not to stay overnight. Again consultants for the same operations may take widely differing times in theatre not least because they either have different techniques or different patient types: with reimbursement of theatre costs now usually based on the category of operation not the time taken in theatre, it is important to have the information systems to monitor this and plan theatre time accordingly.

Supplies

The importance of proper management of supplies increases as the industry moves away from the 'fee for item of service' or 'cost plus' system of billing. However in most hospitals the ratio of supplies sales to supplies costs still remains an important statistic in assessing the adequacy of revenue capture and mark-ups have historically been generous. Hospitals have also in the past opted for disposable and therefore chargeable rather than reusable items to boost revenues especially as there are no established guidelines as to what medical and pharmaceutical supplies should be used or charged to the patient: consultant preference still plays a major role in the former.

Some hospitals charge for the majority of supplies individually: in addition to providing valuable cost profiles, it can substantially boost revenues but over-zealousness may cause adverse patient and insurer reaction especially in respect of items of small value whose external prices are readily available.

At the other end of the scale hospitals without management information and stock control systems may prefer a more limited range of often inclusive charges, such as an all-inclusive theatre pack charge: this has the benefit of simplicity but may, without regular review, lead to under-recovery owing to the higher than average inflation rate for medical supplies. The middle ground is to record all material items used for costing purposes but to leave the decision whether to charge to the business office. It is administratively simpler to charge a higher mark-up on high value items that a lower mark-up on everything: the cost of recording the charge for a tongue depressor, for example, is unlikely to be recovered. Similarly the recording of the right number of units is critical: unit dosage and charging are especially difficult for items such as fluids and many hospitals have prospered from charging for a partially used full bottle.

It is essential that methods of charging, either by charge sheets or peel-and-stick systems, are comprehensive and fully understood and adhered to by those responsible for charging (usually department staff): this includes proper notation of quantities and units of charge. Many medical staff will be unaware of the cost of supplies that they use with a tendency, intensified by deep feelings that it is wrong to profit from illness, not to record charges. The proper use of coded charges even in a manual system will avoid incorrect charging by accounts clerks who will usually be unaware of commonly-used alternative name and standard dosages.

Good supplies management lies also in the minimisation of stockholdings and efficient buying policies. Again it is essential to employ the right person for a small but specialised and often ignored department. Larger hospitals or groups of hospitals can achieve appreciable savings by bulk purchasing and stock transfers between hospitals: these savings may be achieved by the smaller hospitals by either confederate purchasing or contracting with the NHS. Buying from a supplies wholesaler is easy for the inexperienced buyer but is not cost-effective as negotiated discounts can be large: too many administrators do not understand and therefore avoid involvement in supplies management.

Minimisation of stockholdings is most easily achieved by strict control over both stock ordering, usually through one point, and departmental issues and stockholding. The last can be achieved through proper monitoring and restocking of fixed departmental or 'par' stocks, not least involving reconciliation against supplies charged. As in other industries ordering must be 'just in time' rather than 'just in case'; and with a large number of items in stock from many suppliers economic order quantities, delivery times, and alternative sources must be established. A hospital's stores, especially pharmacy, will comprise a mixture of essential fast-moving items and slow-moving items, often with expiry dates. To be successful, minimisation of departmental stocks must be accompanied by a department's trust that stocks will be available when required: a department will otherwise maintain its own reserve stock.

The change from the cost-plus system has, as noted above, diverted the materials management mentality from efficient cost recovery systems to efficient cost management. The argument between disposable and reusable has arisen again, over-prescription is being curtailed, and the best buys are being sought often in the face of consultant conservatism and disapproval. This is especially so in the case of generic drugs where low cost is set against perceived quality. In this as in other areas it is only a knowledgeable manager and peer pressure that can counteract a consultant's knowledge and habit.

Medical fees

Medical fees relate primarily to the need for a qualified medical interpretation of certain tests — for example pathology tests, X-rays, electrocardiographs (ECG's), and health screening assessments. Surgeons' and anaesthetists' fees, when included in a hospital bill, are usually excluded from both revenue and expense. The most common ways of paying medical fees are by either a fixed annual sum (with or without incentives) or a fee for each item of service which may be simplified into a share of departmental revenue or even profit. The relative merits of each depend on the expected utilisation of a service (a fixed-sum contract may be advantageous for an expanding department but not for a declining one) and the perception of the doctor's role in expanding services. In all cases the costs can be high if badly negotiated: for example a consultant radiologist may commonly earn anywhere between 20 per cent and 40 per cent of the department's revenue. It is important to remember that the doctor as an individual may have a widely different view of the financial arrangements from the hospital as a corporation.

Subcontracted services

We have already spoken about the advantages and disadvantages of subcontracted services. There can be no hard and fast rule, a decision being dependent on the skills available to a particular hospital and its catchment area, the maturity and occupancy of the hospital, and the perception of its role and function. For a mature and complete hospital it is usually true that the provision of services in-house is cheaper, more efficient, and easier to control, especially in revenue-earning departments. There are additional benefits in team-building and consistency of quality and corporate culture.

Overheads

Although the above are the major costs for a hospital, proper cost management can also significantly affect other areas such as utilities, repairs and maintenance, insurance, marketing, office administrative costs, and property and finance costs. Control of these costs is often ignored or inadequately delegated. It is essential that each cost is made the responsibility of a departmental manager and is subject to a higher review.

The importance of a budget

A well-prepared and monitored budget is critical in controlling both costs and overall performance. This should normally include projected monthly profit and loss accounts for each department, balance-sheets, and cash-flow statements, with working capital, cash-flow, and capital expenditure as well as profit and loss and statistical targets properly monitored and incentivised. Since its reasonableness will be heavily dependent on achieving expected occupancy levels it is essential that this area is well-researched and co-ordinated. It can be achieved by a review of historical seasonal fluctuations in admissions and likely future holiday periods (consultant, patient, and public), consultant research and interviews to establish their likely future practice, and co-ordination with marketing and capital expenditure plans.

Hospitals differ over which revenues and costs, especially overheads, should be allocated to particular departments. Some costs, such as depreciation, can be specifically, even if not usually, so allocated: but such allocation will not significantly improve budgetary control while less scientific overhead allocations are usually misunderstood and divert attention from the costs that are really controllable at departmental level. Some services — health screening is a good example — use the services of more than one department and their revenue is thus often split. It is suggested however that most revenue and cost allocations conceal rather than reveal and are unnecessary if budgeted and actual performance are consistently compared and responsibilities properly delegated.

Revenue and occupancy budgets are usually prepared in some detail on a monthly basis. The commonest mistakes on the cost side are either not to flex costs at all in line with revenue or to assume that they flex fully. Both assumptions are unrealistic. Easy access nowadays to microcomputers for budgeting purposes makes sensitivity analysis and realistic flexing of costs possible for even the smallest hospital.

Capital expenditure and growth

Expenditure on an existing facility

Private hospitals require continuous reinvestment to replace old or obsolete equipment, to acquire new technology, and to maintain the interior and exterior fabric of the building. Reinvestment at a level exceeding the annual depreciation charge is not uncommon with critical reinvestment decisions usually encountered five to seven years after opening as initial equipment becomes outdated.

Equipment

Major reinvestment in equipment requires detailed research into its feasibility on a payback, profitability or cash-flow basis. Replacement may be essential to maintain medical standards, while investment in new equipment may, even if viewed in isolation as a loss-maker, have wider implications in attracting new consultants and services. Consultant preference, expertise, and projections of utilisation will also need critical assessment. Radiology, for example, is often quoted as a department which is unlikely ever to make a net profit after proper allocation of equipment financing and maintenance charges but which is usually essential to a hospital.

In reviewing investment decisions, management must first be clear of a hospital's long-term strategy — is it to specialise and invest in high technology or remain the general hospital of tradition? To be in the vanguard of medical technology, be it lithotripsy, CT scanning, transplant surgery, cardiac catheterisation and angioplasty, or nuclear magnetic resonance (NMR) may be a substantial marketing weapon in the short-term but competition, limits in the availability of relevant medical expertise, and the sharply-falling price of technology may often alter projected utilisation and profitability. The cost of a CT scanner, for example, has fallen by up to 75 per cent in the last five years. The initial expense of treatment has also made insurers, with their actuarial premium calculations historically based on 'cold' non-emergency surgery (with major surgery performed in the NHS), shy away from extending cover unless there are proven savings in the cost of treatment. Smaller hospitals, incapable of considering such investments, have sometimes lost market share but have often retained more profitable low-acuity business and have attracted back those surgeons who have felt excluded by the increased specialisation of the major hospitals. The surgical procedure most commonly performed in a private hospital remains the removal of impacted wisdom teeth.

Buildings

Expenditure on existing buildings can be split in two: expenditure required to maintain the fabric of the building, normally a profit and loss item; and expenditure on internal reorganisation and restructuring especially when combined with an overall building expansion programme, normally a balance sheet item. Although there are no industry-specific guidelines or recommendations, the accounting treatment of such expenditure may be critical to its feasibility and profitability. Increasingly hospitals follow the example set by hotels and offset expenditure on building maintenance against regular asset revaluations.

Although investment in relation to turnover is high and technical obsolescence quick there are no UK industry guidelines on recommended depreciation lives though they are available in the United States. Consequently different companies have widely different policies which blur direct comparison whether for competitive or acquisition analysis. Many hospitals have followed the lead of the hotel industry in not depreciating buildings and have further treated 'fixed equipment' (such as lifts, piped gas systems, incinerators, and plant) as buildings rather than equipment.

Hospital profitability would certainly be hurt were an inflation accounting methodology to be reintroduced which valued the depreciation and financing costs of assets at current cost. The timing, cost and location of a hospital investment has always been critical to its profitability and inflation accounting would give too little credence to this: it would however prompt many in the industry to consider seriously whether they are really in the business of property investment or commerce.

Extensions to an existing hospital, given that there is land available, are a cost-effective way of increasing capacity. Investment in additional beds need not entail commensurate investment in other departments such as theatre, pathology, or radiology. The long-term nature of such projects makes proper financial review critical especially where space is at a premium and other areas must be reduced in capacity by internal reconfiguration. It will be important to make a long-term assessment of the interrelationship of the various departments not least the fast-changing relationship between theatre and bed capacity. The shrewd administrator will try to minimise present expenditure while keeping open all future options for further reconfiguration at minimal cost.

Expansion through acquisition or development

Capacity will always place severe limitations on a hospital's earnings growth, and a hospital that ceases to grow is in danger of stagnation. If the possibility of on-site expansion is either unavailable or exhausted then growth can only be sustained by the acquisition or construction of new hospitals.

The decision between construction and acquisition has largely been a historical one. At first construction was the norm as new locations, not covered by an existing hospital's catchment area, were sought and modern hospitals built. The maturation period of new hospitals is long — anywhere between two and five years. Heavy financing costs, low initial occupancy, and the inability to offset large tax losses are a major strain on cash-flow, if the hospital is not part of a large and wealthy group, and are usually underestimated. Those players who entered the development field late are often still struggling to reach profitability.

This, combined with the increasing national coverage of hospitals, has led to the second and continuing stage of hospital acquisition as both a defensive and aggressive strategy. As noted earlier, this is a reflection of the maturing of the industry into separate groups of major and niche players. The relative cheapness but long maturity and higher risk of a development must be set against the higher price but immediate potential profitability of an acquisition.

A successful hospital acquisition will usually require a proper property valuation but the assumptions behind such valuations are often misleading. Original or replacement cost is obviously an indicator of value but an open market valuation, given the small size of the industry and the relative infrequency of hospital sales, is often difficult. Following the lead of the hotel industry, it has been common to attribute value on a price per bed basis. Whilst a good guideline, this will often inadequately account for different levels of equipping. An independent professional valuation, while taking account of the above factors, will usually use the method of capitalising earnings, whether historical or, more dangerously, future. It will also tend to be over-optimistic in attributing an alternative use value. It would not be easy to convert a hospital into a hotel: it has yet to be tried.

Too many hospital purchases have been justified on a low perceived price per bed but have been dependent for future profitability on inadequately researched occupancy growth. Yet the tendency to over-value the investment value of a hospital (a problem even more acute in the nursing-home industry, where the ratio of turnover to investment is even lower) has meant that a reasonable price may often be paid for a hospital only if it is underperforming. The recent accounts for one London hospital with a £6 million turnover incorporate an open market valuation of assets of £30 million. This may reflect London land values but it certainly does not reflect the hospital's earnings: a reader of the accounts should realise that, far from the hospital being successful, its site could more profitably be sold — a good example of the industry not having decided whether it is an investment or commercial operation.

Such valuations are useful for the accountant. Goodwill arising on an acquisition can often be offset by a property revaluation: a policy to allocate such revaluation reserves primarily against buildings, and subsequently not to charge depreciation, is an additional benefit. It is interesting to compare such treatment against the present vogue for valuing brand names, usually also on the basis of capitalised earnings, and thereby perhaps distorting the true purpose of the balance sheet. The only difference for the hospital industry is that it has tangible assets to which it can allocate such valuations.

For both acquisitions and developments a properly constructed and researched feasibility study is essential where projected occupancy will be the key sensitivity factor. A five-year study for a new development may be too short a period given its maturity curve — historical performance may make this realistic for an acquisition — while a ten-year study, in an industry of rapid changes and technological improvements which is unexpectedly different now from what it was ten years ago, may be unrealistic.

Even in the short term, doctors' projections of utilisation tend to be over-optimistic: at the very least their perception of a 'heavy' surgical workload is very different from the hospital's corporate perception. In the long term they must be viewed sceptically and independently checked against other occupancy guidelines. All too often the tendency is for long term projections for different hospitals to look remarkably similar with general experience of positive occupancy growth at other hospitals substituted for a realistic assessment of the specific hospital's potential.

Sources of finance

This disparate nature of the financial structures and ownership categories within the industry make an assessment of the preferred means of raising finance difficult. Bank loans, intercompany loans, both interest-bearing and interest-free, and internal and external leasing arrangements both for property and equipment have been regularly used to supplement equity: even donations to charitable hospitals have either financed investment or subsidised patient care. Such arrangements reflect the interests of different holding companies and cannot be used to establish best practice for the industry as a whole.

However, since tangible assets are the bedrock of a health-care investment, secured bank borrowing is an effective means of financing a hospital, and even more so a nursing home, acquisition. High gearing at an established and profitable hospital when interest rates are low can substantially improve the return on equity but can otherwise be a high risk. Such gearing has never here reached the levels found commonly in the United States because of both historical City ignorance of the industry and the reduced marketability of hospital investments.

For a hospital development, even with substantial bank borrowing underpinned by assets, the long path to profitability, working capital requirements, and pre-opening costs require a substantial equity commitment. Early hospital developments were often either sponsored by doctors or sought doctors' equity participation as a means of underpinning projected occupancy. But doctors, although often fiercely protective of 'their' hospital, make their profits from their fees rather than their investment — in many cases they would be happy if the hospital just broke even — and have usually been subsequently bought out by hospital management groups, a process made easier by ethical guidelines issued by the General Medical Council restricting undisclosed investments of this nature.

Finance has also been successfully raised through BES schemes but recent limits imposed on the amount of such investments and the purpose to which it can be put have effectively now excluded this avenue. Without careful planning and control over performance a venture capital investment can often be upset both by the length of time required for a hospital to reach maturity and the limited exit routes. Leasing of equipment, especially major items, remains attractive to some but has been made less so by the removal of first year allowances.

Internal controls

The basic financial accounting systems, whether computerised or manual, required in a hospital are simple and standard to most industries — sales and purchase ledger, payroll, nominal ledger, and stock control — but must be adapted to reflect the industry's particular needs. On the sales ledger side both the price and the debtors' masterfile ledger will be large. The payroll system is complicated only by the complexities of pay rates in a 24-hour 7-day a week professional environment, but benefits greatly from an efficient labour management and reporting system.

It is not possible to provide definitive guidelines on best practice for the financial controls required in a hospital: that depends on the size of the hospital, the financial awareness of departmental managers, and the role of senior management. The prime areas to be addressed, as for most businesses, are revenue capture, cost management and authorisation, and treasury management. The reporting systems should be designed to ensure that complete information is provided promptly and regularly to facilitate corrective action.

Revenue capture

In comparison to a hotel, a hospital too often seems unable to produce a bill, or at least a complete bill, prior to a patient's departure. There are reasons — a higher number of charges from a greater number of departments in a hospital, less set times for admission and discharge, staff embarrassment in raising financial matters at either admission or discharge, the large number of brief and inexpensive outpatient visits, inadequate business office staffing, and the lack of proper admission and pre-admission procedures — and they are not helped by poor hospital design which has often ignored financial requirements.

Many hospitals send bills out after a patient's departure to ensure completeness of charging: perhaps realistic and appropriate for insured patients where there is less requirement for an immediate bill, it puts strains and cost on the subsequent task of charging, billing, and collection. The patient needs to be educated to expect to pay a bill, unless directly reimbursed by an insurance company, at the time of treatment; and the hospital should develop systems to ensure that an accurate bill can be produced at that time.

In a computerised environment, charges may be recorded centrally or by department: a manual system will usually require the former, on information provided by the department. Although both can work well it is suggested that departmental charging is rarely seen by a department as its prime responsibility and is often therefore inaccurate, delayed or both. Proper procedures for revenue capture, including a complete understanding of what items are chargeable and daily feedback to and reconciliation by department heads, are essential.

Cost management and authorisation

The key question to solve is the level to which the approval of expenditure can be delegated. With so many small departments, often inadequately trained financially, full delegation may lead to lack of control especially for critical issues such as capital expenditure and equipment maintenance. Insufficient delegation will clog the workload of the small number of senior executives — the administrator, the matron, and the financial manager — and, as in many other areas of the hospital, may prevent proper segregation of financial responsibilities. A proper but simple documentation of delegated authority, limited both financially and by expense classification, can be adjusted for each hospital's needs with departmental managers limited to approving or requesting expenditure for their own department only.

Treasury management

Efficient collection of debts is a necessary concomitant of prompt charging. Often ignored, it can only be managed properly by the delegation of specific responsibilities and strict procedural guidelines. The high level of insured business means that bad debt levels are usually low — Central London, with its high level of overseas patients, requires additional diligence — but slow collection can be difficult to correct and has significant cash-flow implications in an otherwise cash-positive industry.

All the components of working capital should be regularly monitored with management ratios. Such ratios should normally include days in debtors, inventory, and creditors, and collection ratios; and a system that facilitates further breakdown of such debtor ratios by payer is invaluable.

Treasury management is very much a monthly cycle. In addition to monthly cash flows being part of the budgetary process, it is suggested that management benefits greatly from daily occupancy, revenue, and cash reports with weekly revisions to profit and loss and cash-flow projections. Receipts and insurance company reimbursement can be estimated with some accuracy and should be synchronised with the monthly payments cycle of salaries and accounts payable. Substantial investment income can be earned from a properly managed treasury function.

Information technology

Cost-effective and comprehensive computer packages are now available to all but the smallest private hospital. These systems can be supplemented by personal computers or manual systems to provide additional management information especially on the costing, labour management, and forecasting side. In an industry that is medically at the forefront of technology and computer engineering both hospitals and insurers have until recently been slow to computerise and had little choice: for the small hospital the purchase and maintenance of American systems has been too expensive and entailed major changes to software that had been designed for a radically different market and reimbursement system. The system now most commonly used is 'Medax', which offers a selection of packages for financial purposes, plus those required for management. It has full UK-based support, and is developing in line with customer requirements. It includes a 'booking' system for reservations and theatre booking, as well as a 'billing' system for patient accounts. In addition it has stores and pharmacy packages, provides statistics and management information, and other functions. On request, the support company will develop other software, either on a custom basis, or with a view to general use, when development costs will be shared.

Given that this system is now the 'industry standard', other companies have really only had the option of offering systems at a more competitive price, but usually offer only more limited systems, or ones that are not entirely proven. Whilst software appears to have become easier to generate, it is a brave company which will take the risk of being a guinea pig in such critical areas.

The ability to analyse the patient and business base can potentially give a hospital a competitive edge, and it is important both to understand the situation relative to competitors, and also to ensure that one's information is as good as that held by the insurers with regard to your hospital — their common practice is to compare costs between hospitals based on various categories of cases, and it is important to have some information to challenge their conclusions.

Unfortunately, many of the management information packages have been developed by people with limited knowledge of marketing, and they have too great a financial orientation. The most useful information is with regard to workload and sources of business analysed by consultant and specialty, and an analysis of GP referrals, to see which GPs are referring, and to whom. There is nothing more frustrating than a computer system which contains a lot of relevant information, but which cannot be accessed.

Great opportunities exist for increased use of information technology. Bar-coding, costing systems, interfaces with medical systems for both charging and medical records or with doctors' offices for reservations, admissions, and the feedback of medical reports, and computerised settlement of bills with insurers are a few examples. The hospital that cannot afford to invest in technology, both medical and administrative, will increasingly find it difficult to remain competitive.

Taxation

Corporation tax

The government has yet to receive substantial corporation tax revenues from the private hospital industry. A majority of hospitals have suffered from initial and often continuing heavy losses, increased by first year allowances on equipment expenditure, which subsequent profits have yet to eradicate except through group-relief schemes. At the same time, with so large a proportion of the industry either charitable or internationally-owned, tax-free status and international tax-planning schemes have reduced the tax payable by the profitable players.

Value added tax

As for many other industries with largely VAT-exempt sales and therefore irrecoverable VAT on purchases, VAT can be a major administrative difficulty and may require negotiation with the Customs and Excise. A small hospital may not reach the levels of taxable sales above which registration for VAT is required — on sales of such items as prescribed drugs, hotel services such as catering, telephone charges, and accompanied accommodation, and consulting room rentals which include secretarial support — but equipment sales may change the position overnight.

Where appropriate, hospital groups have tended to obtain group registration to avoid unnecessary losses on intra-group transactions but have thereby ensured higher prices to the patient (albeit by a small amount) and a significantly increased administrative burden to account for essentially immaterial amounts of tax. It is difficult, for example, to differentiate not only prescribed against other drug revenues but also the associated input tax: and, since VAT accounting will largely be on a memorandum basis with costs booked on a tax-inclusive basis, computerised accounting systems may require extensive updating for no commercial return.

Previous ways of recovering VAT, either by being part of a non-exempt group, by manipulation of the ratio of input to output tax, or by the establishment of non-exempt, such as intra-group leasing, companies, have largely been eradicated by recent changes in VAT legislation which have required matching of inputs to outputs. In addition recent legislation to introduce VAT on new construction has made hospital growth more expensive.

Annex: Financial support for patients from public funds

Paul Ridout

This annex looks at the financial support of patients by the government. Public funds may be available to support the care of patients in private nursing homes from two sources:- the District Health Authority (DHA), and the Department of Social Security (DSS).

The District Health Authority

The role of operating a free National Health Service imposed upon the Secretary of State for Health by Parliament is delegated to the District Health Authority (DHA).

In appropriate cases a DHA may elect that care of patients within its district be provided by contract with the private sector. That is a matter for direct negotiations between the private sector supplier and the DHA so as to identify the service to be provided and the price to be paid. The matter will be conducted at arm's length between the negotiators on either side. A detailed examination of such negotiations is beyond the scope of this section.

The Department of Social Security

Parliament has enacted that public funds be paid as a matter of right by the Department of Social Security (DSS) to those of insufficient means to provide for their own needs. In most cases the entitlement to such funds is a matter of right derived from fixed statutory provisions which provide no great flexibility in any direction. Such payments include supporting the recipient in residential accommodation which he requires but cannot provide from his own funds and, where nursing care is required, may include support for that prospective patient towards payment of his fees at a nursing home.

The benefit was originally called Supplementary benefit and until 29 April 1985 was paid to the full extent of the charge made by a nursing home provided that the nursing home was providing care and making a charge reasonable in all circumstances. However after 29 April 1985 such support has been limited and the policy of limitation is now to be found in the present law where the payment made is described as 'income support' identifying its true nature, i.e. a support to the patient towards fees rather than a grant to discharge total fees.

An understanding of the limitations and operations of the system for claiming and receiving income support is vital to the administrator of any nursing home.

Source material

Social Security Act 1986

This is the principal statute from which the entitlement to income support is derived. Any detailed examination of a case will probably turn upon the interpretation of the regulations made by the Secretary of State under the Act.

Income Support (General) Regulations 1987

Social Security payment regulations are constantly subject to review. This section takes account of amendments up to and including the Income Support (General) Amendments Regulations 1988. In considering an individual case one should always make sure that no additional regulations have been made and it is vital to consider the original regulations rather than the resumes issued by the DSS whether in their so called 'yellow book' or otherwise.

Social Security (Claims and Payments) Regulations 1987

These regulations lay down the rules for making claims and the times when payments of benefits shall be made. Understanding these rules is vital in advising prospective patients and their relatives of the steps which they have take to make a claim. A prudent nursing home manager will not admit a patient to a home in the knowledge that the patient is dependent on Social Security Benefit until satisfied that a claim has been made and accepted.

Who may claim?

The fundamental rule of income support cases is that the support is paid to the applicant. The nursing home is not entitled to any payment and has no position in the making of the patient's claim save for providing supporting evidence. If the patient is not in a position to deal with his own affairs or to understand procedures it is possible for him to have an agent know as an 'appointee'. The appointee will normally be the closest convenient relative or possibly a friend or neighbour. An appointee may be a representative of the nursing home. Practices differ but many Departments of Social Security are curiously opposed to the appointment of a nursing home manager as an appointee; some on the contrary welcome it. The majority practice is not to permit nursing home managers to be appointees unless there is a total shortage or lack of willingness of any close relative or supposedly independent person to undertake the role.

This is curious because the sole role of the appointee is to make an application in which he will be wholly dependent on information supplied by the nursing home and then to collect payments, if the application is successful, and distribute those payments for the benefit of the patient. In effect this means that the whole payment will be made to the nursing home.

If an appointee is involved, nursing home managers should ensure that they have a proper contract with that appointee to ensure payment and monitor the contract to make sure that payments are made regularly. There have been a few cases (only a few) where appointees have misappropriated funds. In such cases the nursing home's remedy lies against the patient and the appointee and there is no right to recoup the money once again from the Department. Vigilance is the watchword.

The home owner must remember that there is no claim for fees against anyone other than the patient or a person who has entered into a contract with the home. No claim will lie against the appointee if he discharges his duty properly. Anomaly may arise on death. It is likely that the appointee will be responsible for the funeral arrangements and may discharge those expenses from his own money. The funeral expenses are a prior charge on the estate of the deceased. The estate may consist only of the entitlement to residual Income Support. In the absence of a contract between appointee and nursing home there would appear to be no reason why the appointee should not use residual Income Support payments to discharge the prior claim of the funeral expenses leaving the nursing home unpaid. The problem may be avoided by contract.

How is a claim made?

A claim is made by the applicant or his appointee to the local office of the DSS upon an appropriate form which will be issued only by the Department. Applicants may find that only one form will be issued when a prospective claim is made.

The information required on the forms is: name and address of the applicant; income and capital of the applicant; and needs of the applicant.

Home owners must make sure before admission that at the very least the claim form has been lodged with the DSS. Under no circumstances will any claim be paid from a date earlier that the receipt by the Department of the form.

When can a claim be made?

A claim can be made when the need arises. An important and little publicised change was made with the Income Support (General) Regulations 1987. For Supplementary Benefit no claim could be made till the patient had taken up residence in the home.

Now where a claimant does not fulfil the conditions for entitlement but anticipates that he may satisfy those requirements within three months, the application may be made and the award will be deferred until the requirements are satisfied. This will clearly apply to an applicant whose capital resources are running out. It also clearly applies to a prospective patient who is not in a nursing home and therefore does not satisfy the requirements for residential accommodation income support but anticipates that he will be admitted within three months.

Home owners are recommended to advise all potential residents who will require income support to deal with the application using the three-month rule prior to admission and then to plan the date of admission accordingly.

From when is payment made?

The earliest date from which payment can be made will be the date when the claim form is lodged with the Department. However there is a hidden trap. Payment will only be made in respect of a benefit week and the first payment will be made upon the first day of the benefit week after the claim is lodged.

The first day of a benefit week is a movable feast. Social Security Benefits are paid from different days of the week. Schedules 6 and 7 of the Social Security Claims and Payments Regulations 1987 must be studied.

If admission is not carefully timed there will almost certainly be a gap which is unpaid. Home owners and managers must ensure that the fees for that gap are provided by payment in advance or by contractual obligation. It does appear that the gap may be made up if the patient is good enough to die early in a final benefit week! Positive planning for admission using the three-month rule outlined above is the real answer.

In emergencies owners must get contracts and preferably payments in advance to secure the position.

Sometimes income support is paid in arrears, sometimes it is payable in advance. This will depend upon the nature of Social Security benefit to which the applicant is entitled. Most support will be paid in arrears but support to those receiving pensions is paid in advance so that for nursing home owners, who largely care for the elderly, income support is payable in advance.

How is support calculated?

Having identified that the applicant needs support the DSS will assess the applicant's resources. The applicant's income and capital will be assessed. Detailed consideration of this is beyond the scope of this section but there are traps. Capital may very well include sums which do not appear obviously as part of a patient's capital. Income may include sums to which the applicant is prospectively entitled although not immediately and obviously entitled as a matter of enforceable contract. Certain resources are disregarded.

Each individual case will turn upon its own facts and the Department will absolutely refuse to discuss the case with a nursing home owner unless he or she is the appointee.

Two important points

Payments by third parties to supplement the shortfall between nursing home fees and income support, i.e. payments by relatives, charities or possibly health authorities or other Government agencies are disregarded. Thus there is no risk of a generous relative's payment working adversely to claw back support.

Capital resources may include resources of which the patient has divested himself unreasonably. This has caused difficulties and in some cases might be seen as conflicting with Inheritance Tax planning. It is more in the nature of straightforward fraud. Relatives may hit upon the idea of persuading their elderly ones to divest themselves of their capital by giving it to younger relatives and then presenting the elderly person as a penniless applicant for income support. Investigations show that where that is the case the claim to support will be rejected. The writer has only discovered this in very few cases but home owners must be vigilant and it is yet another reason for making sure that the Income Support claim has been processed and agreed and is in a position for payment before admission, i.e. use the three-month rule!

What is the maximum level of support?

The maximum level of support is set out in Schedule 4 to the Income Support (General) Regulations 1987. In difficult cases the Schedule must be studied.

The maximum level of support is the actual charge to the claimant or the upper level specified in the regulations whichever is the lower.

Two important points arise:-

i. The maximum fixed arbitrarily is the maximum charge considered to be appropriate, i.e. the maximum charge if the claimant has no resources. If the claimant has resources which fall to be deducted they will be deducted from the maximum. In the standard case of a general-nursing-home patient the maximum level (currently £190) will be reduced by any retirement pension or other Social Security benefit, e.g. attendance allowance payable to that patient.

It is not £190 plus the benefits but rather the reverse *plus* the personal allowance often nicknamed 'pocket-money'.

ii. If the charge is lower than the maximum the claimant is obviously only entitled to the charge made. The claimant is to be supported and no profit is to be made from support.

Personal allowance or pocket-money is payable to the claimant as with all other benefit and/or support and there is no restriction on the way in which the claimant should spend that personal allowance. Provided that the claimant understands what is happening there can, it is suggested, be no objection to the pocket-money being used to assist in defraying excess nursing home charges.

What is the maximum will be in many cases a subject of lively debate with the DSS.

Nursing homes are not registered by District Health Authorities by reference to the categories of income support, listed in the regulations.

District Health Authorities are not concerned in the level of benefit payable to patients and should not interfere. The DHA will have registered a nursing home with or without categorisation of patients. That Certificate delimits the category of patient for whom care may lawfully be provided. The intention of the Certificate is not to delimit the levels of benefit payable. If a patient category is specifically excluded (and only in that case) not only will an enhanced level of benefit not be payable for the patient at the home but it is illegal for the home owner to keep such a patient in the home. The two prepositions are inseparable.

The problem will arise where patients are diagnosed as physically disabled or terminally ill and more frequently in the latter case.

With effect from April 1989 patients in this category are entitled, if in receipt of appropriate care, to a maximum of £235 per week support.

General nursing homes may lawfully care both for the physically disabled and for the terminally ill. The legality of care is determined by the Certificate of Registration. Health authority officials who suggest that benefit is not payable in respect of a patient apparently entitled to a higher level must be prepared, if they intervene (and they are advised not to intervene), to justify the proposition that placement of that patient in the particular home is unlawful and home owners are recommended in those circumstances to require the DHA to take responsibility for the patient and place him or her elsewhere.

Physically disabled patients are only entitled to higher-level benefit if they were physically disabled prior to pensionable age. Homes for the young physically disabled will have all patients entitled to higher level of Benefit if they qualify otherwise by reason of the care provided but should remember that their benefit is payable in arrears rather than in advance. Physically disabled patients over pensionable age may be entitled to an enhanced claim only if they are able to prove that they were physically disabled prior to pensionable age and that may be difficult to prove.

There is no definition of physical disablement within the 1987 Regulations. I would suggest that physically will be interpreted as distinct from mentally and that disabilities should be given a wide construction to include any impairment from normal function.

Terminally ill patients have more frequently experienced problems. Development of the hospice system and the specific development of special techniques to care for the dying or the terminally ill have clouded this issue. Terminal illness has been defined as an illness where the medical prognosis leads to recommended treatment changing to palliative from curative. Nursing homes are registered to care for the sick and that is clearly indistinguishable from the ill. Whether an illness is terminal is a matter of fact to be shown by evidence supported by the expert evidence of doctors and nurses involved with the patient. A patient diagnosed as terminally ill by his or her doctor is entitled to receive the benefit at the higher level.

That is not an end of the matter, two further points arise:

i　Higher benefit is payable only if it is shown that the care provided for the patient is consistent with the higher level of dependency, i.e. a terminally ill patient must be shown to receive care appropriate to the terminally ill. Diagnosis of terminal illness is not a terminal bonus in Income Support terms for the nursing home. Greater dependence leads to greater nursing care requirements which cost more money leading to a higher charge to the patient who in consequence is entitled to expect higher level support to meet the additional cost.

ii　The home must charge the higher cost if there is one. If no extra charge is made the DSS will rightly reject a claim for enhanced benefit for the maximum claim is the charge made by the home. It is folly to support the patient in making the claim without additional charges having been made and then expect the claim to be backdated. The writer knows of no commercial disadvantages in raising invoices for nursing-home fees (which do not attract VAT) in advance of determination of the claim. If the claim is rejected after Appeal the nursing home is still entitled to expect to be paid but may of course on commercial grounds decide to waive the extra charge. That is a matter for the nursing-home owner.

The nursing-home owner will undoubtedly be called upon to support the patient's application. The following procedure is suggested:

i　The patient's condition is identified as terminal.

ii　The nursing-home owner requests a detailed report from a responsible doctor outlining the condition and the prognosis.

iii　The nursing-home matron assesses the condition and reviews the patient's care plan.

iv　The nursing home manager reports the position to the patient or the patient's relatives and indicates that if the patient is to remain in the nursing home additional fees will be chargeable, but the additional support may be available.

v　Claim for additional support is lodged upon the first day of a benefit week.

vi　New care regime is implemented.

vii Details of the diagnosis, the change in care plan and the care provided are submitted to the DSS together with the increased charges.

If that procedure is followed there should be no difficulty in obtaining payment.

Bridging the gap

In most cases there will be a gap to be bridged. There is no discretion in the Department to make increased payments. Other sources must be found. The most common are charities providing for the elderly, and the patient's relatives. The nursing-home owner must ensure an enforceable contract for the duration of the stay at the nursing-home to pay the additional sum by a third party. Without a contract the third party may change their mind at any time.

There is much debate as to whether health authorities can be a third party providing the gap-bridging payment. There is nothing in the Social Security Act 1986 or associated regulations which prevents that course. District Health Authorities are entitled to enter into contracts with nursing homes for the provision of care for patients within the responsibility of the Authority. Some Authorities will suggest that the legislation governing their administration and application of funds prevents making the so called top-up payments.

There seems to be no convincing argument to support this and it is likely that health authorities' unwillingness to make top-up contracts is grounded in a commercial decision not to enter into long term commitments rather than any legal inability.

Patients in nursing homes before 29 April 1985

When the cash-limiting legislation was introduced it was recognised that this could cause hardship to patients already in nursing homes and accordingly provisions were made to protect the level of their benefit (now income support).

This protection is often misunderstood. Before 29 April 1985 there was no limit on the amount of benefit payable. Now there is always a limit. The limit for pre-1985 patients is the amount of the charge made for the nursing-home accommodation in April 1985 plus £10 or the aggregate of the estimated reasonable charge for a nursing home in the same geographical locality and providing the facilities the claimant requires plus £26.15 plus the applicable amount of the attendance allowance if the claimant is so entitled, whichever is the lower.

In practice the better alternative is likely to be the former. The significance of this provision will evaporate. The number of pre-1985 patients will diminish and the maximum levels of support have been increased over subsequent years and no doubt will be increased in the future so that slowly the maximum support payable will inevitably exceed 1985 weekly charges.

Whether or not the maximum level of support can be increased is entirely at the discretion of the Department. The Department will have to decide whether or not the protection is required to avoid exceptional hardship. That is at the discretion of the Department and is not subject to Appeal to a Social Security Benefits Appeal Tribunal. Clearly the Department must act fairly in exercising its discretion.

A problem arises in proving the existence of exceptional hardship. Clearly the prospect of eviction from an established nursing home is exceptional hardship. However as the maximum level of support is still limited, if it be the case that the increased payment will not meet the nursing-home charges the hardship will not be avoided. If a claim is to be made for this extra amount it is vital that the nursing-home owner agrees to accept that increased amount in discharge of the patient's obligation or, if that is not shown, the Department will say, quite correctly, that the hardship is not avoided so that additional payments should not be made.

4 Caring for the patient

Sally Taber

Anyone who has worked in health care knows the importance of nursing. Without the support of caring and professional nurses the sector could not exist. Almost everything we do by the way of delivery of health care depends on the nurses. Our success is dependent on their contribution and support. Both managers and doctors recognise their importance. This chapter covers their role, and the ways in which we can support and develop that role.

Background

Nursing in the private sector has been considered as either pandering to the needs of the wealthy in a private London hospital or caring for the elderly in a nursing home. It is hoped that the following chapter will convince you that neither assumption is correct.

The independent health care sector is mushrooming. The market analyses since 1979 suggest a trend towards profit-making beds with fewer charitable beds available. The independent sector, therefore, endeavours to attract nurses who demonstrate a commitment to developing themselves both clinically and professionally. This should ensure a sound foundation, for the building-up of private health care in the UK.

A commitment to a high standard of service and client satisfaction is required of nurses who wish to practise in the independent sector. Such traits as empathy, care and compassion, should be included among their interpersonal skills. We are willing to further develop such traits and qualities in the independent sector, and through our training and education programmes, this is already paying dividends in terms of patient care.

It is imperative that the nurse caring for patients in the acute private hospital has the support and confidence of the multidisciplinary teams. She acts as the link person for the consultant. He depends upon her integrity and professional judgment in the absence of an established medical infrastructure.

The nurse learns to manage her time more effectively. The emphasis is placed upon 'quality time' with individual patients, as the majority of patients are in private rooms. How do nurses know that the patient is safe and comfortable and how do very busy nurses give the patient the impression that they have all the time in the world for them yet still leave the room after an appropriate time without leaving the patient feeling abandoned?

Nurses have to develop this skill rapidly, as well as enhance their powers of observation to identify when the patient wishes to be left alone. Active staff development and continuing education are required to ensure that nurses in the private sector meet these specifications.

Continuing education and staff development

A definition of continuing education is important because it provides a frame of reference on which to build. A useful working definition is that of the American Nurses Association

> *Continuing education in nursing consists of those planned educational activities intended to build upon the educational and experimental bases of the professional nurse for the enhancement of practice, education, administration, research or theory development to the end of improving the health of the public. (1984)*

Education should be seen as a continuum, and inherent in the philosophy underlying the preparation and role of the practitioner must be commitment to the concept of progressive and continuing educational opportunities throughout the career of the individual. Such opportunities must be available to all nurses in the private sector. The main goal of continuing education should be to improve the individual's level of competence through enhancement of knowledge, skills and attitudes in a variety of settings at different points in the practitioner's career, thus ensuring high standards of patient care. It should give the practitioner confidence, job satisfaction, and the ability to adapt to new approaches and also provide help in change of career direction.

Because of the lack of a traditional educational infrastructure within the private sector, clinical credibility has been adversely affected.

How have we in the acute-care setting altered this perception?

Expenditure on nurse development and post-basic education

Intravenous workshops are provided in which counselling is given — counselling to reach the required standard of competency. The general aims of the intravenous course are as follows:

- That the nurse should gain a deeper understanding of her/his professional role when preparing and administering intravenous drugs.

- That the nurse should become safe and competent in the preparation and administration of the above drugs and is aware of the importance of maintaining accurate records.

- That the nurse should gain an insight into the pharmacological aspects of drug administration, to ensure the safety of the patient.

  Other internal courses are:

- Controlled drug update for Registered and Enrolled Nurses.

- Clinical developments e.g. wound management and infection control updates.

- Safety aspects: lifting techniques update, sharps/hepatitis update, advanced cardiac life support and ECG workshops.

There is a designated person to attend to the above needs and identify positive career routes for nurses in the private sector, while measures to promote staff development include:

- Commitment to study leave both internally and externally and the recording of such experiences in a specially designed booklet.

- The awareness that working in the private sector, can sometimes lend itself to professional isolation. This can be overcome by a formal link with a NHS College of Nursing.

- The encouragement of all levels/grades of nursing staff to actively participate in in-house seminars/lectures. To develop teaching/communication skills so that nurses' knowledge and skills can be imparted to their colleagues in a professional manner.

Project 2000

The nurse in the private sector must be aware of the implications/ramifications of Project 2000. How can this be achieved? Some suggestions are:

- Promoting day release for degree/diploma studies.

- Identifying the sisters/charge nurses in need of teaching and assessing skills, secondment on ENB 998 courses.

- Identifying the need amongst all nursing staff that 'Mandatory Updates' will be a prerequisite for continuing nursing in the 1990s.

- Assistance offered to our Second Level Nurses on the road to conversion by undertaking ENB 933 courses (Professional Development Course for Enrolled Nurses) and receiving tutorial support from a recognised College of Nursing to satisfy ENB requirements. There is a need for accurate profiling of all members of the Registered/Enrolled nursing staff to identify deficits and future developmental requirements.

- Staff must be recruited and retained in the light of demographic changes in the early 1990s. Assistance should be given to those members of staff who do not want to convert to RGN status.
  Assistance is also needed by those nurses who may wish to 'return to

nursing' after a break of five years or more. Such requests can be facilitated by offering the ENB 902 course (Back to Nursing).

The industry as a whole will have to look positively at job sharing, and other flexible arrangements if it is to achieve staffing targets over the next decade.

• The controversial role of the Support Worker requires urgent examination in the private sector. Aspects include: safeguarding standards; implications of paying for care, but receiving 'hands-on care from an unqualified person'; competencies designed by whom, monitored by whom; liabilities rest with hospital director/director of nursing? We need to involve ourselves in the current discussions and ensure we are keeping abreast with the current recommendations and the National Vocational Guidelines being recommended.

Feedback is the life blood of learning, therefore a formally organised appraisal system described later in the chapter permits the individual to identify his/her own educational and development needs. It provides the opportunity to negotiate learning — in post-basic education. It should be non-threatening, for the well-being of the nurse and discuss an awareness of career development.

The ethos should NOT be to keep the nurse at any cost, which is detrimental to the nurse, but also eventually to patient care. Rewards should be not solely in financial terms but also in personal professional development.

All such courses — as well as the external conferences, seminars, specialist updates — promote a sense of confidence in nursing practice. Caring for patients can therefore be undertaken against the backdrop of up-to-date knowledge and skills, ensuring that the right attitudes and behaviour are displayed at all times, because.....

'People are Patients: Patients are People'

Criteria for learning environment

A philosophy of care for the floor/department/nursing home with clinical learning objectives and expected outcomes should be established. It should include the following aspects:

• Adherence to hospital policies such as: infection control, drug administration and lifting techniques.

• Annual staff appraisal and three-month post-probationary period appraisal.

• Adequate supervision of new members of staff using an induction programme. Establishment of a mentor system in each area to ensure the nurses' individual needs are met.

• Regular unit meetings to ensure that the clinical environment is continually evaluated. The establishment of a safe working environment with all the relevant mechanical aids and equipment.

- Regular updates in advance cardiac life support (ACLS), fire drills, drug administration and lifting techniques.

- Access to appropriate visual aids/library facilities and journals to maintain professional knowledge and skills.

- Appreciation and application of nursing research to clinical practice.

Philosophy of post-basic nursing education

Post-basic nursing education (Princess Alexandra College of Nursing) is based upon the belief that education is a lifelong process, and is the responsibility of the individual. The nurse is encouraged to develop through clinical practice an up-to-date knowledge of the skills required to care for patients and their families who require specialist nursing intervention. The emphasis placed upon self-directed study is directly related to the nurse's motivation, to maintain his/her clinical expertise, and demonstrate at all times the use of professional judgment to promote optimum standards of patient care and safety using assessment planning, implementation and evaluation of nursing actions. Such actions will be based upon the designated model of care. This emphasises the activities of daily living and patient dependency criteria. Whenever possible such practice should be based upon nursing research. The nurse should be aware of his/her role as patient advocate, and as therefore primarily accountable to the client for the delivery of specialised care.

The provision of a positive atmosphere for professional development, assists the nurse in broadening her knowledge base and places his/her skills and attitudes in a dynamic continuum.

The philosophy of care within the private sector should not differ. An example of establishing a philosophy is as follows:

Each patient is a unique individual, whose rights, customs and beliefs must be respected at all times. Each individual has a right to health, based upon biological, psychological and social continuity of well-being.

The nurse should assist the patient and his family, at all times, to satisfy his/her health-care needs, to regain independence and control over his/her individual health care.

The designated model of nursing with its emphasis on assessment, planning, implementation and evaluation of the individual's activities of daily living should be used as a framework to achieve a biopsychosocial balance and continuity of well-being.

The enrolled nurse

The independent sector, by definition, endeavours to be a profit-making entity, therefore we cannot afford to lose our Enrolled Nurses — we must invest in them. It is important that we offer them professional development and post-basic educational courses (McGuckin, 1989).

Many more doors of opportunity will be opening for those Enrolled Nurses who have specialist experience, evidence of professional development and a commitment to their professional status. Conversion is not the panacea for all. I would suggest that we as educators and managers have an obligation to provide Enrolled Nurses with the appropriate knowledge and skills, so that the choice for conversion will be made in the light of knowledge, rather than the fear that they might become obsolete.

Clinical auditing

The preparation of an audit is essential within the private sector and should be part of the licensing authority's check. It enables the nurse to ascertain the cost of the care to be delivered and to ensure that the floor/ department/nursing home is living within the budget. The degree of accountability that nurses are required to exercise nowadays should be stressed. Clinical auditing perhaps acts as a tool in this respect. It certainly places the onus on the managers to ensure the clinical environment permits the safe practice of nursing. Another benefit is that the qualified nurse can refer to the audit as a measure of potential learning opportunities, as well as a bench-mark for required standards of care.

Clinical auditing areas that should be addressed are:

• Nurse establishment
• Ratio of trained nurses or ratio of appropriately qualified staff in specialist clinical field
• Skills identified
• Skills mix
• Clinical activity
• Communications
• Learning climate
• Mentorship
• Teaching staff
• Physical environment
• Nurses' perceptions of the learning environment

Performance appraisal

Performance appraisal within the private sector is well-defined and well-documented because of the need to perform to the highest possible standards within financial constraints. Recruitment is expensive so that it is essential that every effort is made to retain staff.

Performance appraisal can be described as the opportunity to:

REVIEW — PREVIEW

LAST YEAR'S PERFORMANCE AND ACHIEVEMENTS

NEXT YEAR'S FORWARD PLAN

Performance appraisal is the systematic evaluation of the individual with respect to performance on the job and potential for development. The most important purposes of performance appraisal are:

- To review current performance by means of a constructive two-way discussion.
- To improve current performance.
- To set performance objectives and standards for the coming year.
- To identify training and development needs.
- To draw up succession plans.
- To motivate and stimulate staff.

Measuring standards of performance

Standards of performance are the measuring or assessing device for the key-result areas or tasks of the job. A standard of performance should state the level at which performance of a key-result area or task is satisfactory.

A standard of performance uses QUALITY, QUANTITY, COST or TIME as a means of measuring. Standard objective measurements are seen to be more fair than subjective measurements but are not always possible.

Criteria for Standards

Every standard of performance needs to be clearly and accurately understood on both sides — by boss and subordinate. Any disagreement at appraisal time over its meaning shows the need to stop and clarify.

Every standard needs a time element built into it — 'how much within what time', 'how many over what period', 'how often by when'.

The appraisal interview

Interview preparation

The various stages are:

1 Gather and collate all the necessary information: job description; personal file; previous appraisal; performance objectives; key tasks and standards; key incidents; and any note you have made during the year.

Table 4.1 Preparation for performance appraisal review by the interviewee

1. What are the main tasks, in order of importance, which you are required to perform?
2. What aspects of your job do you do best?
3. What aspects of your job do you do least well?
4. What have you accomplished during the last 6/12 months?
5. With regard to your present job, what do you hope to accomplish over the next 6/12 months? (Wherever possible, please give measurable objectives with a time limit.)
6. Do you think that you have a complete understanding of the requirements of your job? If not, of what are you unsure?
7. Are there any problems outside your control which have reduced your ability to perform your job?
8. What training do you think would help you to perform your job more effectively?
9. Do you have any skills or talents which are not being used to the full in your present job?
10. Are there any parts of your job which you think should be altered in any way for any reason?
11. Is there any particular career within the organisation which you would like to follow if you were given the chance?

Table 4.2 Points for satisfactorily conducting an appraisal interview

1. Create a relaxed, informal atmosphere.
2. State objectives of the exercise.
3. Explain the procedures involved, i.e. forms etc.
4. Explain how you wish to conduct the interview.
5. Get the employee to assess his performance first.
6. Use open-ended questions to get a discussion going.
7. See whether details are missed or the interviewee speaks in generalities.
8. Ensure your review covers all the key areas of the job, the standards and any short term priority tasks.
9. Make your assessment known to the person.
10. Discuss any points arising from your assessment.
11. Praise work well done.
12. Point out areas for improvement and the reasons why.
13. Demonstrate how you think these areas can be improved.
14. Encourage
15. Summarise from time to time.
16. Get employee to give views on his future development.
17. Discuss future training needs and development.
18. Finalise the discussion by a quick overall review of the interview.
19. State what will happen to any action plans, i.e. attendance on a course.
20. Show what will happen to the notes taken.
21. End the interview on a positive note.

2 Plan the interview. Decide how you are going to handle it: the major points you wish to raise about performance, the target areas and objectives you wish to agree for the future. Consider what problems may arise during the interview.

3 Give the interviewees time to prepare, and ask them to prepare some notes on their perception of their own performance. Guidelines for the appraisal such as those given in Table 4.1 can be helpful.

4 Do not fill your day with a stream of appraisal interviews — they take time and energy. It may be the interviewee's sole opportunity to have your individual attention for any length of time.

5 As far as possible arrange in advance not to be disturbed during the interview.

6 Avoid undue formality.

7 Be at the appointed place at the appointed time and be prepared.

Time management

Providing care in a high-dependency environment places demands upon the effective use of time by the nurse.

The nurse is made aware of principles in the context of time available, and meeting deadlines. Emphasis is placed upon setting and meeting objectives/targets, and being directly answerable if they are unmet within the given time.

Quality care can be given in quality time. This principle applies to us in all areas of our lives but especially in the private sector where for most of us the demands and pressures on our time greatly outweigh what is available.

By making more effective use of time the nurse will not only gain more control over her job and her life, but she will accomplish more of what is important to her.

The following is an example of a Time Management or Improvement Programme (Bremner):

CONTENT
Identification of key areas and activities of the job.
Planning: setting goals and priorities.
How to manage interruptions
How to control and prevent crises.
Making meetings effective.
Delegation.
Other time management aids or techniques.
Developing a personal strategy for the future.

To obtain maximum benefit from the course, participants are asked to undertake the following pre-course preparation:

1 Identification of priorities and key areas of their job;

Breathing
1. Unable to maintain respiratory function without mechanical assistance.
2. Respiratory function maintained through an endotracheal tube/tracheostomy, ability to clear secretions not fully effective.
3. Respiratory function maintained with oxygen, physiotherapy or drugs.
4. Requires some preventative assistance to maintain normal respiratory function.
5. Able to maintain normal respiratory function without assistance.

Consciousness
1. Requires continuous monitoring, does not respond to painful stimuli.
2. Responds only to painful stimuli, neurological observations remain unstable.
3. Requires drug therapy to control confusion due to neurological disorder.
4. Requires neurological observation to detect/prevent deterioration, no confusion evident.
5. Patient is fully orientated in time and space, no assistance required.

Circulation
1. Intravenous (IV) drug intervention and mechanical ventilation required to maintain adequate circulation.
2. Adequate circulatory function maintained by IV drugs.
3. Oral drugs used to maintain adequate circulatory function.
4. Only monitoring to detect potential deterioration in circulatory status required.
5. Circulatory function maintained without assistance.

Safe environment
1. Unable to maintain a safe environment, totally dependent on nursing intervention.
2. Can maintain a safe environment but requires assistance most of the time.
3. Can maintain a safe environment, requires assistance occasionally.
4. Can maintain a safe environment, rarely requires assistance.
5. Able to maintain a safe environment without nursing intervention.

Mobility
1. No spontaneous movement, requires total nursing intervention.
2. Limited spontaneous movement, requires assistance to change position.
3. Can change position but requires assistance to mobilise.
4. Requires encouragement/teaching to mobilise.
5. Can mobilise freely without assistance.

Hygiene and skin care
1. Totally dependent upon nursing intervention to maintain hygiene and skin-care needs.
2. Limited ability to care for hygiene and skin care, requires nursing intervention most of the time.
3. Requires assistance to care for hygiene and skin care needs.
4. Only requires assistance occasionally to meet hygiene and skin-care needs.
5. Able to maintain hygiene and skin care needs without nursing intervention.

Eating and drinking
1. Requires total parenteral nutrition.
2. Enteral feeding and/or hydration with IV fluids required.
3. Requires help with eating and drinking, possible intermittent enteral feeding to supplement.

4. Requires assistance with eating and drinking and information and teaching re special diets.
5. Can maintain own nutrition and hydration unaided.

Elimination
1. Intermittent/continuous renal replacement therapy required.
2. Catheterised and requires intervention with drugs to maintain diuresis and requires bowel management for constipation/diarrhoea.
3. Catheterised, but only requires assistance to use bedpan/commode, drains in situ unproblematic.
4. Requires teaching re diet and fluid intake to maintain adequate elimination.
5. Needs no assistance with elimination.

Rest and sleep
1. Requires continuous strong sedation at all times.
2. Requires strong sedation only at night, to sleep, reduction during the day to rest.
3. Only requires sedation at night to sleep, rests well during the day.
4. Requires a warm drink and quiet environment to rest and sleep.
5. Requires no assistance to rest/sleep.

Knowledge skills
1. Lacks total knowledge and understanding, requires full training/educational programme by nursing staff.
2. Small amount of knowledge, needs further education/clarification by nursing staff.
3. Knowledge and skills being gained, requires guidance from nurses and family.
4. Sound knowledge and skills, sometimes requires occasional assistance from nurses and family.
5. Full understanding, knowledge and skills achieved, no need for nursing intervention.

Social/cultural
1. Totally dependent on nursing staff to satisfy social/cultural needs.
2. Nursing staff primarily responsible for satisfying social/cultural needs with occasional help from family, friends.
3. Joint responsibility for helping to satisfy social and cultural needs held by family, friends and nurses.
4. Able to satisfy own social/cultural needs with help from family, friends and occasional nurses.
5. Able to satisfy own social/cultural needs.

Psychological
1. Totally dependent on nursing staff for satisfaction of psychological needs.
2. Nursing staff are primarily responsible for satisfying psychological needs with occasional help from family, friends and religious personnel.
3. Nurses, family, friends jointly responsible for helping to satisfy own psychological needs.
4. Able to satisfy own psychological needs with help from family, friends, minister and sometimes nursing staff.
5. Able to satisfy own psychological needs.

Communication
1. Unable to communicate verbally or non-verbally.
2. Unable to communicate verbally due to endotracheal tube/tracheostomy in situ.
3. Can communicate non-verbally, but has difficulty speaking the language.
4. Can communicate verbally and non-verbally but with some difficulty.
5. Requires no assistance with communication.

Table 4.3 Criteria used for nursing assessment

2 Identification of main time-management problems at present; and

3 Analysis of current utilisation of time by using a time log.

Patient dependency

A system to assess patient dependency helps ensure that the patient numbers are equated with the cost of nursing time. It is essential to measure the dependency of the patients in order that the budgeting process and hence the cost to the patient can be accounted for. The checklist shown in Table 4.3 provides an example of the criteria used for nursing assessment and for measuring patient dependency.

Measuring patient dependency

Having set out in Table 4.3 some basic criteria, it is not an easy task to create a general model for measuring patient/nurse dependency in a high dependency unit.

Three main elements of data must be collated: regular patient dependency categorisation; levels of nursing staff per shift; and sampled observations of nursing time devoted to patients in different categories. Collection of these data would enable the average nursing time for a patient to be calculated.

A problem with taking sampled observations of nursing time is the difficulty of measuring anything other than time spent directly with the patient. Indirect nursing time cannot easily be attributed to a specific patient.

An accurate method of categorising patient dependency is set out in Table 4.4.

Patients in category A usually require a nurse ratio of 1.5:1. These are the most seriously ill patients and need a greater degree of nursing care and attention. It is recognised that a single nurse will be unable to meet all the patient's needs during the course of a day. Situations may arise when a patient is compelled to return to theatres for an emergency procedure, or the patient may have a cardiac arrest. Contingency plans must be available to ensure that nurses can maintain the care of the remaining patients in the department.

Medium-dependency patients (Category B) usually require a 1:1 nurse ratio while for the low dependency patients in Category C a 0.5:1 ratio should be adequate.

Theatre nursing

Many independent hospitals have been purpose-built to incorporate state-of-the-art technology in conjunction with pleasant surroundings. In this acute-care hospital, great emphasis is placed upon meeting the needs

Table 4.4 Categories of dependency [in a H.D.U.]

Category A (acute or high dependency)

Cardiovascular:	Cardiac instability or poor cardiac function such as cardiac arrest, acute dysrhythmias, e.g. balloon pump or lotochemotherapy support. Heavy blood loss 7150 mk/hr.
Respiratory:	Requiring mechanical support or when 'weaning'.
Renal failure:	Such as acute renal failure (together with respiratory support).
Neurological:	Deep coma, no reaction to painful stimuli, no gag reflex (together with respiratory support).
Metabolic:	Instability, such as acute crises, i.e. hepatic coma, diabetic coma, gross electrolyte imbalance.

Category B (medium dependency)

Cardiovascular:	Adequate cardiac state, infrequent or stable chronic dysrhythmias; minimal cardiac support; minimal blood loss.
Respiratory:	Self-ventilation with some support; may require suctioning and have tracheostomy.
Renal:	Improving or steadily changing condition requiring dialysis on alternate days, continuous peritoneal dialysis or haemofiltration.
Neurological:	Deep coma including some response; gross confusion.
Metabolic:	Impaired liver function, portal hypertension; controlled diabetes on sliding scale insulin.

Category C (low dependency)

Cardiovascular:	Stable cardiovascular state — no support.
Respiratory:	Self-ventilating with oxygen.
Renal:	Satisfactory renal function — no support but may be catheterised.
Neurological:	Drowsy but rousable, mild confusion.
Metabolic:	Controlled diabetes, stable electrolyte balance, satisfactory liver function

of the consultant users, and accommodating their requests for specific equipment or investigations.

This approach to customer care is also adopted in the theatre environment and the (consultant) surgeons negotiate with the senior theatre nurse for appropriate operating slots. The senior nurse is responsible for liaising with the reservations department, to ensure that the patient and consultant have a mutually agreeable time for operating. It should be emphasised that delays or cancellations of surgery do not often occur, since the consultant is allocated space for a specific length of time, and is therefore accountable to one of his colleagues if he/she 'overruns'.

The skill mix in this particular theatre setting is varied, and the close working relationship that exists between the first and second-level nurses and the ODAs fosters a good team approach. The basic theatre team consists of: one to scrub; one to circulate; and one to assist the anaesthetist. A flexible approach to working hours is encouraged, and flexi-time has been incorporated into the system. Meeting the demands of the consultant users, and being adaptable is an integral part of theatre nursing.

The on-call team are responsible for dealing with surgical emergencies during the night, and the theatre team have to be prepared to undertake bookings at unsocial hours.

The opportunity for theatre nurses to assist the surgeon in doing a 'list' does not often rise. The nurses have to liaise with several different surgeons/anaesthetists in perhaps four theatres simultaneously, and they must be aware of their idiosyncrasies.

The opportunity to develop both clinically and professionally is improving rapidly. The introduction of quality circles and setting standards is now under way. The organisation of consultant lectures and seminars is encouraged. The nursing staff are liaising with the ODAs in training staff and attendance at external seminars is considered imperative. The formal links already established with a London teaching hospital have afforded us (at the London Bridge Hospital), the opportunity to share knowledge and expertise, and reduce the feeling of isolation that can frequently arise in such a specialist sphere.

The independent sector realises that theatre nurses are at a premium and that therefore it must demonstrate a commitment to in-house training and skill development. The introduction of comprehensive induction programmes and an established Mentor system is now under way.

Teaching and assessing courses are offered to senior nurses so that their role as facilitators/mentors is enhanced. The development of pre- and post-operative visiting must now be considered an integral part of the theatre nurse's role.

The cost-effective management of such a busy and diverse department requires further training on the part of the theatre superintendent. Each staff member is made aware at the monthly meetings of his/her responsibility for cost-effective practice whilst ensuring patient safety at all times.

Infection control

Infection control is as important (if not more so) in the private health-care sector as it is in the NHS. The users of private health care, i.e. consultants and patients would be quick to go elsewhere if a private hospital had a reputation for poor infection control. Scrutiny of the private sector by public bodies is more intense than in the NHS because we have no Crown immunity from the Health and Safety Inspectorate and furthermore we have to be registered with the local health authority who come to inspect our premises twice a year.

Aspects of infection control are present in all hospital activities e.g. bedside care practices, theatres, CSSD, handling of clinical waste, catering and food hygiene, laboratories, engineering and plant maintenance and of course, housekeeping. A further aspect in London hospitals, and some peripheral hospitals dealing with acute patients, is the care of patients from overseas who may present special infection risk problems.

Who carries out infection control? Usually a nurse who has been given a certain amount of training in infection control protocols, but it is usually only one of her roles — she may also be a floor sister or departmental manager. As in the NHS it is recommended that she works with a doctor employed by the hospital to be infection-control medical adviser and the infection-control nurse liaises with all relevant departments, particularly the laboratories.

The main activities should be 'trouble shooting', helping to devise systems and working practices and most importantly education and training. The latter function is made easier in the smaller hospital units and better communication is found in the private sector, also funding for education and training is more generous.

Finally an obvious advantage for the private sector in maintaining high standards of infection control is the larger number of single-patient rooms with private bathrooms and high housekeeping standards, all helped by being set in modern, high quality, easily and well maintained buildings.

Organ donation policy in the private sector

Introduction

Organ transplantation depends on the altruistic willingness of people to help their fellow human beings.

Donation provides the donor family with a means to assist others, and also to alleviate their grief in the loss of a loved one.

Most acute care private hospitals are rarely in the position of admitting trauma victims. Therefore, should a death occur in the hospital, it may well be unexpected and would probably be a result of unforeseen surgical complications.

Realistically the majority of the patients treated within an acute-care hospital will not be multi-organ donors because of the lack of trauma admissions. Even so, most can be potential corneal donors. Whatever the 'gift', the relatives have the right to choose. Effective and efficient mechanisms are essential if potential donors are to be identified and organs and tissue retrieved in a timely and dignified fashion and then transported to places in which they can be used appropriately.

It has been shown that a significant impediment to organ and tissue retrieval is the lack of an established system in hospitals for identifying and referring potential donors.

We have identified a need at the London Bridge Hospital, with its multiracial and multi-religious patient population, for an established policy of organ donation and retrieval which can be tailored to the hospital's involvement and circumstances, and is consistent with regional policies.

Any health care professional can identify a potential donor. Staff who are uncertain about the suitability of a potential donor should contact the hospital transplant co-ordinator. Should he or she not be available, then the regional transplant co-ordinator should be contacted. No potential donor should be deemed 'unsuitable' until one of the above has been consulted.

Perfusible organs may be obtained from donors pronounced dead on the basis of neurological evidence, but with respiratory circulatory function maintained.

Death can be made manifest by irreversible cessation of the functions of the brain, or of respiration and circulation

Brain-stem death means the clinical absence of brain-stem function, defined as profound coma, apnoea and the absence of brain stem reflexes. Brain death signifies the death of a patient, but respiration and circulation can be supported to maintain organs until removal for transplantation.

The diagnosis of brain death should be made by, or in consultation with, physicians experienced in the required examination, and familiar with the accepted criteria. No physician or surgeon who may be involved in the care of a potential recipient may be involved in the brain-stem assessment. These tests should be performed individually by two separate clinicians, one of whom must be a consultant neurologist.

The Coroner may have to be consulted, particularly with patients who died within twenty-four hours of having surgery.

Role of the transplant co-ordinator

He/she will co-ordinate the approach to the family, and liaise with the nursing and medical staff regarding the donor maintenance and care prior to removal of organs. He/she will directly contact the regional transplant surgeon on call in the case of kidneys, and ophthalmology hospital in the case of corneas. He/she will notify the regional co-ordinator of the situation, enlisting their help, in the case of a multi-organ donor, in contacting the team concerned, retrieving the organs, i.e. heart, lung and liver, and subsequently in handing over the responsibility for distributing them to the regional co-ordinator.

Approaching the family about donation

Foreign nationals dying in an acute-care hospital should not be considered as potential donors unless their families offer spontaneously. This has been decided in view of the differing cultural backgrounds and the possible problem of misinterpreting the hospital's motives for seeking organ donation by the patients' families or the Embassy sponsoring them. This statement is constantly reviewed depending on attitude changes.

Families of patients resident in this country may be approached provided the consultant's approval has been outlined. If the family spontaneously ask or request donation, then the consultant should be informed of their decision and the co-ordinator may proceed.

The hospital transplant co-ordinator is available for twenty-four hours a day, providing assistance and advice. If for any reason he or she happens to be absent, then the regional transplant co-ordinator is to be contacted.

The cost of procurement of organs is identified and passed on to the appropriate recipients after approaching the family about donation.

It is essential to remember that tragedy occurs in the private sector and that out of a tragedy can come some good.

Co-operation with the NHS

What can we learn from each other?

Quality of service, analysis of past performances and cost effectiveness are common themes within the independent sector. Why can't we share our expertise in such spheres with our nursing colleagues in the NHS? We both operate under strict financial constraints; therefore the development of interdisciplinary courses, open days and shared resources can guide us towards the 'same purpose' — improved patient care. A cross fertilisation of ideas amongst nursing professionals promotes a deeper awareness of the problems facing nurses in both sectors.

The private sector must recognise the need to further the development of clinical learning environments so that nurses from the NHS may gain knowledge and skills in a different philosophical setting but with the 'same purpose' — to deliver the best care to a patient whenever and wherever needed.

Professional associations

There is a risk of professional isolation within the relatively small private units and involvement in external professional activities helps keep one up to date. 'Inform' and the IHA act as the two best points for professional contact.

INFORM— forum for independent nurse managers

Inform provides nurse managers with access to the Royal College of

Nursing (RCN). The aim of the forum is

1 To encourage membership growth within the independent sector and encourage participation by independent sector members in the activities of the RCN at all levels, in particular to encourage members who are eligible to participate actively in the activities of INFORM.

2 To raise the profile of nursing and nurses in the independent sector, in particular to enhance the public relations role of INFORM with the media generally and the professional journals in particular.

3 To facilitate increased understanding and joint professional activity between the NHS and the independent sector.

4 To assist in the development of effective and efficient management practice within the independent sector by professional education activities and information sharing.

5 To assist in the development of nursing practice and nurse education within the independent sector.

Independent Hospitals Association (IHA)

The role of this association has been described earlier in the book. The part of the IHA pertaining specifically to senior nursing personnel is the Nurses and Training Committee. It has as its brief:

1 Scientific input for the Annual IHA Conference

2 Liaison with the English National Board

3 Planning of Regional Meetings

4 Liaison with Inform

5 Production of a Training Guidelines Folder and a Central Training Register.

The Committee is also responsible for forming local membership groups and assisting them in achieving its documented objectives. The main reasons for establishing local membership groups are:

to discuss issues of concern within a local labour market; to consider information and initiatives from IHA; and to ensure the IHA Nurses and Training Committee has direct feedback from the membership and discusses issues of concern to the local groups.

It is worth mentioning the importance of both Inform and IHA working together on certain points and being complimentary to each other.

Nursing home environment

It is essential that a patient being cared for within the nursing home environment is assured of high standards and that the nursing staff are accountable for their practice.

A checklist prepared by Lewisham and North Southwark Health

Authority (see Appendix l) provides useful guidelines to ensure that this does actually happen.

Conclusion

This chapter is intended to highlight how nursing in the private sector has 'come of age'. The birth and infancy were troublesome and the child often misunderstood. Now in the light of recent social and political developments, health care in the private sector has become a credible and reliable alternative to the NHS.

I do not underestimate the need for constant vigilance, and have therefore emphasised the importance of professional development and continuing education.

Other private sector health care establishments will differ greatly from my clinically acute environment, but I feel that the principles outlined in this chapter can be applied in all situations in which patients depend upon nursing intervention.

References

Bremner M 1987 *Performance appraisal.* St Martins Hospital Training Document

Bremner M 1988 *Time Management.* St Martins Hospital Training Document

English National Board 1986 *Continuing education for nurses, midwives and health visitors: Stage 1* May

Hartley-Cooper J 1987 *Organ donation policy.* London Bridge Hospital

Lewisham and North Southwark Health Authority *Expected standards to be achieved and maintained in registered private nursing homes*

McGuckin C 1989 Enrolled nurse in the independent sector. Paper presented at RCN Seminar on the Professional Development of the Enrolled Nurse: February 1989

Nursing Standard 1988 Spreading the benefits. In search of the 'perfect' nurse. Who owns what? In Independent Sector Supplement 26 November

Princess Alexandra College of Nursing *Philosophy of post-basic nursing education*

Acknowledgements

Grateful thanks and appreciation are to be given to: Clare McGuckin, Education Officer; Marjorie Bremner, Group Training Officer; Lynne Cleland, Theatre Superintendent; Jane Fawcett, Infection Control Sister; and Michael Bell, Deputy Director of Nursing, all of London Bridge Hospital, for their assistance with this chapter.

5 Staffing

Robin Scott

Health care is a major employer, and the staff are a crucial element in the organisation. We chose to specify the term 'staffing' rather than 'personnel' to emphasise the practical aspects. The writer has rightly looked at the whole area of human involvement in the organisation, and emphasises that staffing cannot be considered in isolation. Our view across all the chapters is that there is a real need to look at the organisation as a whole, with a recognition that all the elements are important, and must mesh together.

Introduction

My reaction when I was asked to write on staffing was that, for me, this represents a narrow but crucial part of the broad range of activities embraced within personnel management, which is increasingly represented as human resources management when operating at a strategic level.

That said, I recognise that readers of this chapter will range from the owner/proprietor of a nursing home or small hospital through to senior executives of major multinational chains, charity organisations, and NHS units. Owners carry much of their strategy in their own minds, whereas executives need to reach agreement with their colleagues before they can jointly engage in the business of directing and motivating the employees.

In this chapter which is broad and general rather than detailed in intent, I shall endeavour:

a) to make a general comment on the contribution of personnel/human resources management;

b) to reflect on some trends in the 1980s and to identify areas of major concern and change in the 1990s; and

c) to offer my views and comments on personnel areas that I regard as critical in achieving effective management within an organisation.

Finally, my colleague Peter Naylor has contributed some notes on the use of psychometric tests in human resource decision making (Appendix 2).

Contribution of personnel (or human resource) management

The Institute of Personnel Management's (IPM) definition expresses the range of the subject (1979):

> *Personnel management is that part of management concerned with people at work and with their relationship within an enterprise. Its aim is to bring together and develop into an effective organisation the men and women who make up an enterprise and, having regard to the well-being of the individual and the working group, to enable them to make their best contribution to its success.*

There has been much recent debate about the supposed differences between a personnel or human resources management approach as to the management of people in organisations. For me, human resources management has evolved from personnel management and includes its objective and its techniques; the shift marks the greater involvement of line management in resolving the human resources question arising when developing business strategy.

Whatever one calls the contribution I have always believed that you can only develop a people-orientated approach through an organisation by embracing the human resource questions within all strategic discussions. The potential contribution of personnel specialists, who have the skills and perception to integrate both strategy and techniques, is brought out for me by considering the concept set out by James J Lynch (1975):

> *'The main power crisis facing modern industrial society is the inability of organisations to release the full potential of people. This inability stems from many causes: badly designed, frustrating jobs; badly structured organisations; outmoded working methods; obsolete machines; restrictive rules of trade unions; suspicious attitudes among both management and staff; inadequate training. Whatever the cause, the effect is the same. People do not give their best and organisations do not reap the full benefits of their manpower.*
>
> *PeoplePower is simply the sum of the knowledge, skills and latent potential of people, individually and collectively. Modern society, through its huge investment in education at all levels, is acquiring greater abundance of human resources than ever before. At the same time, there is an increasing awareness in industry that people are not making available anything like their full capabilities. This discrepancy between actual and potential achievement is what we have chosen to call the PeoplePower Gap.'*

Clearly this situation is wasteful and potentially costly; each and every day an organisation loses potential profit and wastes valuable resources. This is illustrated in Fig. 5.1 which is taken from Lynch's book.

The obvious implications are that the daily waste of potential and resources is great and the people policies are crucial. The employee contribution needs real acknowledgement not just in an annual report but in the daily realities — in creating the 'climate' and style most likely to motivate that makes the difference between mediocrity and excellence in organisational performance.

D

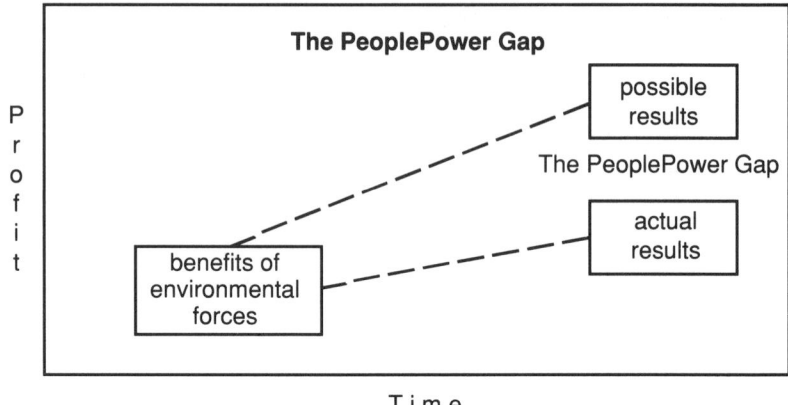

Figure 5.1 The PeoplePower Gap

Human resources management can offer the key to balancing organisation and people interest so that policies and practices are aimed at and achieve 'competitive advantage' for both. In many young or start up operations this level of operation has not been reached or recognised and where specialists exist they are 'tied' to limited areas such as staffing and training. Success comes from integrating human resources into policy and decision making at a strategic level rather that in a piecemeal introduction of personnel management techniques to meet particular problems.

To move from organisation-wide issues to the individual, we need to consider motivation. Clearly we can study behavioural science research and use such ideas as Maslow's hierarchy to talk about the various influences on individual work behaviour but for me it is a manager's ability to focus on the mutual interests between organisation and individual and to communicate their relevance to each member of staff to gain their commitment. Motivation is the driving force that makes the difference between an involved, satisfied, outstanding contributor and a discontented individual who may well be disruptive.

Given the significance of people in providing services — and as a cost — within hospitals and nursing homes, I believe the personnel management contribution in business planning and the expression of it in identifying, nurturing and releasing employee capabilities, is the only way the PeoplePower Gap will close (and thereby increase profit, charitable surplus or simply improve all services to the benefit of all).

Development and training needs

It has been a decade of growth, through new building, natural growth and, more recently, by acquisition. Beyond this basic 'unit' growth there has been a growth in the range of services. All this has meant a pressure on people resources and I would say diluted skills in some key areas. Quality control, although another pressure, is essential and will ultimately prove advantageous to all who work in the sector or use its services.

It seems to me that only the larger companies have been able to move beyond the commissioning/opening preoccupation to develop their climate and framework to the point where they are satisfying their own resource development needs. The 1990s will see further pressures from the market-place which I believe will mean fewer larger groups and even more emphasis on a 'people-oriented' approach.

Human resources management (HRM) is still evolving in the private health sector and is only generally practised and recognised in the bigger organisations at the present time. The smaller organisations need to rely on their luck with their leaders. If I were asked to choose the area of HRM in which most benefit could be reaped for effective management of hospitals and nursing homes in the 1990s, I believe that area would be training and development at every level. There used to be an excuse and fear that if you trained people others would benefit; now, if you do not train you will not attract and retain staff.

On the training front, with the exception of a few very notable cases, it seems to me that the private sector has been very blinkered in its approach to training. A few major organisations have developed sophisticated development programmes for their staff and have reaped the reward after a number of years. Some organisations, particularly psychiatric services, have developed very useful links with the NHS and with the medical professional bodies in trying to develop a joint approach to training. I believe these efforts will have to be magnified very considerably to meet the significant pressures in the 1990s arising from demographic changes and increased mobility of staff.

The search for highly skilled business men and women who can act as hospital directors and directors of nursing has been increasingly difficult because there has been a lack of training within the sector overall and a lack of commercial experience within the pool from which these people are most regularly drawn.

Organisations are now looking for people to lead their units who can be strategic in their approach to the development of business activity for this and the next few years and at the same time are capable of meeting individuals and relating to their particular needs for their own development and future. This dualism will, I believe, be the essential hallmark of the effective manager in the next decade.

The determination of staffing in the early 1980s was dominated by relatively inflexible labour management techniques. I believe there is more flexibility in addressing these issues now, more consideration of activity levels and certainly much more involvement of staff in considering what is possible. The battle for staff, and that is how it might be, is more intense in London and SE England but will be a problem everywhere with fewer school leavers being chased by more organisations than every before.

The employment climate, particularly in the private health sector, is currently threatened with major change because the NHS White Paper suggests a very considerable possibility of market forces rather than state public ownership and bureaucratic procedures dominating the situation. It is probable that private employers will no longer be able to have some fixed relationship with the pay and benefit scales and practices of the NHS, they will have to think for themselves. Pay and benefits in whatever organisation we are talking about — charity, company, residential home or private hospital — will need a radical review.

Finally and most significantly, nursing will be the major issue for the 1990s.

The sector faces a recruitment crisis and much energy will be expended in determining how different skill levels can be used to meet the variety of needs in the different units. The efforts of Project 2000 and perhaps the introduction of a care-support qualification, are just two of the interesting developments now that will affect the 1990s. Training is also emphasised again when one considers the mandatory updating for certain professional health care qualifications.

Recruitment and selection practices

The recruitment of key executives and specialists is one of the most critical activities of directors and senior management. It is expensive (if a proper evaluation of the time and effort put into the exercise is made) whether undertaken by the company itself or by an outside consultant. Within health care there are special areas where shortages of skills make it particularly difficult to find suitable applicants or to properly sustain a service, thereby affecting the basic business capability.

So where do we begin the business of finding the human resources to fulfil an organisation's goal? I believe that it is imperative to start with the question 'is the job really necessary?' I say this because recruitment is often undertaken for a replacement without a check on the changes that have occurred or the skills available in other people within an organisation before embarking on an expensive and time-consuming outside effort. Internal solutions or reorganisation may offer a swifter, cheaper and internally supportive solution. Could the duties be reallocated? Could the vacancy be used as a development post so that a person without the full skills could gain experience for broader benefit at a higher level?

Criteria for selection

Let us assume such checks have been carried out and it is not possible to reallocate duties or to use it as a training post. The next critical step is to ask what are the criteria for selection to the post? To many people it is a surprise to be asked this. I have been asked to find — say a hospital director — and told ' You know what we want, find one for us'! It may be true that I have a general idea of the sort of criteria that might be used but I cannot take for granted the nature of the job, not least because I have to look for the candidates' interests as well. I need to know in considerable detail about the company profile, job accountabilities and work relationships.

It is even more important for the organisation to be clear about what is really wanted. Are the priorities changing between the characteristics that they seek? It never hurts to review the job description or the key tasks that are currently being undertaken by key people against known plans and foreseeable changes. It is essential to undertake this review so that the job and person specification can be developed; only then can a thorough job be done in seeking suitable candidates for interview. From another point of view, perhaps more defensive, it is interesting to note a recent tribunal case (Dr Noone v N W Thames RHA) which identified the lack of clear selection criteria as a reason for accepting a claim of discrimination as justified.

Recruitment

Given a clear brief on what we seek, how do we find candidates for the job? We can consider: advertising, the most frequent medium for communicating vacancies; local agencies; consultants in the case of senior jobs; registers or even outplacement consultants. For general staff recruitment an alternative is to invite staff to introduce suitable people, often in connection with an incentive scheme, or use personally delivered letters to all residents in an area. An efficient personnel department will usually be able to contact people who have left to follow up previous casual inquiries. Increasingly companies are building contacts with schools and colleges as the threat of increased competition in the 1990s comes nearer. Press advertising is still the main medium, with radio and TV being the greatest communicators (at the same time the greatest administrative headache if they are used). This takes me on to the next point that I should like to make.

The administration related to a recruitment exercise is significant; it gives a candidate a picture of the business he/she is dealing with. Is it swift and efficient in its contact or is it slow and cumbersome? Is it informative or is it an organisation that needs pushing to give out information? Before interviewing, preparation is essential. Has the interviewer a frame of reference for collecting information from any discussion that takes place? Does he or she use the C.V. or application form or any letter that the candidates have provided, to make a decision? How is extra information gleaned from the conversation used? What matters is that there should be a systematic means of gathering information that can develop clear criteria for the job and a person specification so that when it comes to choosing between people, information is gathered against this frame making quite clear the objective grounds upon which the decision is being made.

The interview

The interview is the most popular mode of selecting people for jobs and is essentially a conversation to determine a person's interest in a job and to assess capability and suitability for the post.

Many interviewers will be reluctant to accept that a decision on acceptance or rejection is often made within a few minutes. It is perhaps easier to accept if we set aside the professional horror of such a picture and emphasise that, having acknowledged this common pattern, efforts should be made to use the interview time to validate the 'decision'. Another finding is relevant — that interviewers choose areas to explore that tend to confirm the original image and give more weight to unfavourable items rather than favourable. More significantly, interviewers give away the 'bias' for acceptance or rejection in the manner that they use towards the candidate (expressed in either warm or cool responses or in talking less).

So what can we do to make the interview an effective stage in the selection process?

First, ensure the criteria are clear and known to all interviewers.

Second, undertake adequate preparation of interviewers, candidates and meeting arrangements.

Third, direct discussions from an opening statement of purpose and approach, through open questions and probes to arrive at a mutual satisfaction of information requirements. Spell out doubts carefully. Listen and watch for congruence between body language, general style and answers.

Fourth, all interviewers review findings against the criteria.

Fifth, undertake adequate reference inquiries and supplementary information checks to test the decision. Keep the candidate in touch with what happens next.

Alternatives

The interview is the most common selection form but what about alternatives? For me the most interesting and effective alternative approach, particularly when looking at specialist and management posts, is the development of assessment programmes — expressing a simulated version of the job — in which trained observers watch how candidates perform against criteria of effectiveness in that job.

Another approach has been to use 'testing' to provide additional information. Tests can be a great aid but need careful planning in their selection, administration, scoring and interpretation by a qualified professional. Tests alone are insufficient in my view. Peter Naylor writes further about this aspect in Appendix 2.

After the appointment

Moving on to the next stage — in caring for your investment — it is essential to follow up appointments with positive help, before joining, on the first day with an induction orientation programme, 'sponsorship' in the early days and a consistent performance review process. All the promises made in an offer situation must be fulfilled rather than creating dissatisfaction because agreements are not honoured. Retention is vital to protect your investment of time, money and effort. It is a continuous job and needs regular attention. It may help you to think yourself into the candidate's shoes. What would demoralise you? What would demotivate you? What would irritate you? If you can translate this into their work situation you will no doubt remove many potential 'turn offs'.

Summary

In summary I would say successful recruitment depends on detailed preparation, thorough assessment and supportive administration. Together, these will ensure that the process enables the organisation to acquire staff quickly and effectively at a minimum cost and with a maximum suitability for their posts.

Performance review

Why should managers be interested and involved in the time consuming and demanding process of appraising every employee's performance at all levels?

For me the reasons are strong and self-evident.

First, after having spent time, money and effort on finding people (or developing people internally) and providing at least basic training in company policies and practices or particular job skills — an organisation should seek to care for its investment. This care is demonstrated in both continuous review and in subsequent training and development activities, quite apart from the general communication process with employees.

Secondly, for all staff and particularly for key job holders, clarity in their accountabilities is an essential prerequisite for achieving satisfactory results, i.e. knowing who does what, when, how and for whom. This will ideally be in the context of a statement of unit objectives and company-wide targets (often called a mission statement). It is useful to add to this the personal agenda for job satisfaction and career development that individuals have and which need to be taken into account. This means that new post holders require joint agreement on both a clear job description and its translation into tasks and standards to be met. Only after these are accepted and understood can they properly settle into a post and contribute in the way they are expected to.

Finally it is inefficient and unfair to operate without goals and standards — the bottom-line results will show the difference. Through the process of performance review, an ongoing dialogue is created about the way work is continuing for an individual or a department and the blocks that exist to the proper achievement of goals. When this is brought together in a 'no surprises' annual review discussion it can lead to a review of department relationships and information blocks or omissions; the approach can lead to the positive development of improvement plans for that individual and for training and support plans, all aimed at yet further improvement in results. By taking this process down to all staff the pyramid of improvement plans and development plans can generally improve the results of the company. The process represents a prime opportunity for a manager to keep in close touch with his staff.

Review systems

During my time within the profession I have seen a marked shift away from personality-trait oriented reviews, to joint-achievement oriented discussions looking at objectives, tasks and standards. A survey by the IPM in 1986 (Table 5.1) shows why companies review performance.

Table 5.1 Why companies review performance (percentages)

To assess training and development needs	97
To improve current performance	97
To review past performance	98
To assess future potential/promotability	71
To assist career planning decisions	75
To set performance objectives	81
To assess increases or new levels in salary	40
Others — e.g. updating personnel records	4

(Source: Long, 1986*)*

One point this table makes is that a minority use performance review in determining salary. I strongly dislike a direct connection, because I do not believe that discussions can be productive if the salary outcome is a focus of attention in a performance discussion.

In developing a scheme it is essential to gain commitment to the principles — the practical shape and training in the skills at the top level and then work downward. At the same time the process of development needs to involve staff in non-threatening discussions to enable ownership to spread through the organisation. I have not mentioned forms and administration because it is clear to me that the forms can be reshaped at any time to meet the changing needs/views of those using them.

The achievement of results is through contact, communication and development of a dialogue that is achievement-oriented and collaborative in nature. I believe it is necessary for the individual process to start with a job description followed by an agreed statement of target, tasks and standards for a period, normally one year, and an overall annual review form to collect data for discussion and this should be available to both parties, albeit probably in slightly different form but covering the same ground from different angles. As a consequence of this process the training and development department should be collecting information on the suggestions for coaching and training in the following review period.

Training and development

Training and development is a very significant function in its own right and through its activities touches on people at work in every level of an organisation. It is capable of having a very significant influence on the performance and standards of an organisation. To quote the conclusion of the National Training Award Summary for Chief Executives:

> *'Training is a business activity. Its objectives are serious and it requires serious management. Training exists to support the business. The business does not exist to support the training. So, inevitably, training is the responsibility of business leaders not just personnel specialists. When it receives proper attention from top management it can assist the strategic development of the business, improve operational performance and help to cope with contingencies'.* (Lathrope, 1988)

Basic approach

A basic approach in an organisation might well cover: introduction and orientation for all employees; training for changes in skills and growth of new skills; the development and support of staff in their efforts to grow; and a means of changing culture and company practices to gain understanding and acceptance before effective implementation.

Beyond these basically understood areas for training, it is important to see that training and development can offer a very significant help to an organisation (especially now that skills shortages are going to get worse) because:

> they can help to draw on those extra resources from each individual for the greater company benefit and for individual satisfaction; they can fundamentally sharpen job skills and individual awareness of company objectives in relationship to their work; and companies which provide support and training and development are particularly attractive to individuals who wish to learn new skills and grow so that the acquisition and retention of staff is much easier than for competitors who are not bothering to offer the same training schemes and support coaching.

The work of the National Training Award scheme is very significant, encouraging organisations in every sector of working life and for every purpose, to compete for training awards. The aim of the award is to identify excellence in training development and practice and to demonstrate the link between such training and improved business performance. This scheme attracted just over 1100 entries in 1987 and 1468 entries in 1988. It seems significant that only eight of the entries were hospitals or other medical units. I would hope to see evidence that the independent hospital sector accepts the challenge to do much more training to meet organisation needs in the 1990s.

Health care situation

I am conscious that a number of major health care providers have steadily built significant training programmes for their staff which on the one hand look at the business needs and provide management skills or technical skills and on the other hand provide individual development programmes for the personal growth of their staff. I have the general impression that training, outside the bigger concerns, has been minimal and mainly related to job skills perhaps, within the commercial sector, but certainly not comprehensive or extensive. Psychiatric hospitals, in particular the charitable organisations, appear to have maintained good links with the NHS and professional bodies and have carried out a significant amount of training. It is understandable that in a decade where so many organisations have started up operation or made significant acquisitions, the emphasis has been on getting going and the policies and practices have not been fully developed.

It is now essential for each organisation to look at its needs for the 1990s because its competitive advantage will depend on the quality of staff it can attract and retain. Training and development will play a considerable part in that particular work. In health care the development of a recognised care-worker qualification and the development of support roles will be crucial alongside the major nurse training task and the general professional update training.

Performance review and in particular the benefits derived in the way of training and development plans were discussed earlier. It is important for somebody to be nominated in each unit to follow up such work. 'Follow up' is the most forgotten activity in business. If only we would follow up our own ideas and aims to full satisfaction we would make an enormous inroad into that PeoplePower Gap!

Counselling

On another level — not as a major item but as one that I do not wish to see become a major one — I wish to draw attention to counselling. It is exceptionally difficult for a manager to give unbiased supportive counselling to an employee because the time and effort are at odds with his priority role as manager for the organisation. Of course managers listen to their subordinates and help them with problems, very often leading them to the right people for full support or the resolution to their problems.

As a consultant looking at a number of organisations, alone or with colleagues, I have often come across problems that need professional help outside the run of business. The resolution of such problems can release the people for productive work again but meanwhile they are deeply affected and their performance is marred. I believe each organisation needs to develop an approach to providing counselling services which suit its resources. The larger organisation may be able to afford an internal counsellor but most organisations — particularly the smaller ones — would find it useful to develop a link with an external service that was available to help their employees confidentially, knowing that they would reap the benefit in terms of an employee who is able to concentrate on the job and give of his best and know that the company was being supportive without being too inquisitive.

Summary

I began by begging the question whether we were talking about staffing or human resources management recognising the differences in perspective of an owner manager and a major organisation.

Human resources management is about people at work. It is about integrating the human resources into the business planning process by taking a look at the implications of business plans for people and ensuring that there is a balance between the threads concerning the levels of staff, the nature of skills, the market situation for recruitment, the pay and benefits situation, the training and development practices and employee aspirations. The objective is to maintain individual skills at the level needed for the activities required to retain or improve the competitive advantage whether it be for profitable return on capital or surplus for charitable work.

Difficulties have been experienced because human resources management is about bringing strategic business development and personnel management together and developing the operational linkages between these interests to achieve organisation and individual goals.

For those concerned with the effective management of hospitals and nursing homes my key message is that effective management can only be achieved through success in collaborating with employees to achieve clarity about the organisational goals and the means of their achievement whilst at the same time recognising each individual's contribution and aspirations whilst working within that organisation.

References

Institute of Personnel Management 1979 *Definition*
Institute of Personnel Management Recruitment Code

Lathrope K and National Training Awards Office 1988 *Training and success*. Employment Department Training Agency, National Training Awards

Long P 1986 *Performance appraisal revisited.* Institute of Personnel Management

Lynch JJ 1975 *The PeoplePower Gap.* McGraw-Hill

Maslow AH 1943 A Theory of human motivation. *Psychological Review* **50**

6 Nurse staffing

Sandra Hallett

Because of the importance of nurse staffing we felt the need to commission this chapter to supplement the comments within the last two chapters. There is a clear trade-off between running nurse staffing at low levels, to reduce costs, and the view that nurse staffing is an investment in quality, and that a higher level of staffing helps give a hospital a competitive edge. The balance clearly lies in the efficient use of nursing time, to economise where possible, but also to allocate nurses as necessary to achieve high standards.

Introduction

'Nursing is expensive — very expensive! As both the demand for and cost of providing health care increases, so those responsible for funding that care are anxious to know that care is being provided both economically and effectively'. So a recent article in the *Nursing Times* (1989) succinctly describes two of the key issues facing health care managers today: nurse staffing and quality of care. Increasingly it is being acknowledged that far from being contradictory and mutually exclusive, these issues are two sides of the same coin and as such are inextricably linked. Both however are complex issues, set in tradition and steeped in custom and practice, but recent and future changes make it imperative that these areas are carefully scrutinised. Outdated and time-honoured practices must be replaced by effective and professional resource management.

As demand for services and patient acuity increases along with client and nurse expectations, as markets become more competitive and costs continue to escalate, so the need for flexible and responsive manpower planning becomes self-evident. Many nurse managers have found traditional staffing models inadequate in meeting the changing needs of the industry, but even so, few have sought new models better able to reflect the nature of today's environment. And yet more is to come — Project 2000, changes in clinical practice and work assignment schemes, along with the full impact of the scarcity of nurses will all have to be faced in the 1990s.

The importance of these factors for manpower planning and resource management is indeed considerable. Nurse managers will need to acquire and develop a range of analytical and problem-solving skills, in order to meet the challenges of the next decade.

The price of perpetuating outdated staffing practices will become increasingly evident in dissatisfaction amongst nurses and impoverished services. In a climate where hospitals in both the public and private sectors will be competing for labour and client markets, it will be those whose long-term planning has addressed these issues, which will be best able to survive.

Planning

A key vehicle within which to consider the impact of these issues on staffing, is the planning process. The necessity of establishing a staffing plan which sets out the structure, numbers and grades of staff, is well understood in the context of commissioning a hospital. However, few managers, it seems, undertake the detailed and regular reviews which are essential to test whether previous assumptions, upon which staffing decisions were originally made, still hold true. The result of this lack of ongoing planning is that nursing departments continue to perpetuate structures and patterns of staffing which have outlived their usefulness and respond sluggishly to current trends. Manpower planning is useless as a one-off isolated exercise. It can only be effective as a rational and regular feature of nurse management.

Establishing a planning process

For many nurse managers the structures, grades and numbers of staff will already be established. Thereafter the commonest form of ongoing staff planning is that which takes place concurrently with the annual budget process. The disadvantage of this practice is that against this setting, the manpower planning process is often over simplistic and inevitably becomes subservient to the budgeting activity.

Manpower planning, though an essential ingredient in the budgeting process, is also a key activity in its own right and as such should be treated as a separate but complementary process.

To undertake a manpower review, the nurse manager must first list the many factors, both internal and external, which affect staffing requirements. Alongside this list, the criteria and assumptions which were the original determinants of the staffing plan should be noted. The final stage is to identify the changes and difficulties with the original assumptions, both current and projected. In this way specific factors which do or will put the existing staffing plan under pressure become obvious and indicate necessary adjustments to the staffing plan.

Factors affecting staffing

External

External factors, though important for staffing requirements, are usually outside the control of nurse managers. It is perhaps because of this that there is a common tendency to overlook them in the planning process and yet the staffing pressures that these factors can induce are considerable. Typical of these factors are: patient acuity levels; length of stay; patient age groups; nursing/medical technologies; occupancy levels; and recruitment trends.

The list is by no means exhaustive but does indicate some of the common external factors which need to be considered and planned for in advance, rather than reacted to once problems have arisen. Clearly a change in one or several of these factors will have significant staffing consequences. These need to be identified and quantified as part of the planning process, so that informed decisions can be taken which will ameliorate the effects of such changes on the staffing plan.

Internal

Internal factors are those which are within the influence or control of nurse managers. Obviously there are many such factors which will influence staffing requirements, for example: nursing skill levels and experience; mix of grades; education and training; motivation and work ethic; architecture and functional layout; support services; operational systems; nurse assignment systems; and nursing methodology and practice.

Nurse managers must not only be aware of the pressure these factors place on the staffing requirements but must develop a process for identifying problem areas and planning improvements. Nursing skill levels, experience and motivation will all affect individual efficiency and productivity. The staff planning process is not the vehicle within which to resolve problems of this kind, these must be tackled via other management systems. The purpose of their analysis in the context of staff planning, is in order to recognise that where such problems exist a fall in productivity and efficiency will increase the perceived staffing requirements. It is common practice to resolve problems of this nature by increasing staffing numbers in response to this perceived need, but this tackles only the symptoms not the underlying cause. The actual need is not one of increased staffing, it is one of resolving the problem of motivation etc. The planning cycle, by testing the rationale behind changes in the staffing plan, signals where problems are being reacted to rather than resolved.

The same can apply with other internal factors such as support services. For example, when it is found that nursing intervention is required on a regular basis in order to ensure that a support service is effective, then requirements for nursing hours will be considerably inflated by factors in no way related to patient dependency and nursing activities. The practice of increasing nurse staffing numbers to compensate is a costly and inefficient use of nursing time, and can have a marked adverse effect on motivation, thus reducing productivity still further.

The planning process, by using critical analysis and problem identification, encourages the discipline of examining the root cause of problems for their impact on efficiency, rather than the practice of reacting to the consequences by increasing staffing levels.

Determining staffing requirements

In order to determine staffing requirements, the nurse manager needs a statistical means by which to convert patient needs into a finite number of hours of work. In the traditional staffing model which is still common within the industry, this conversion is achieved by applying a predetermined norm of nurse to patient ratio. Thus a 1:5 ratio produces a need for 4 nurses per shift for 20 patients. The advantage of this method of calculation is its speed and simplicity, however, the disadvantage is the disregard of patient acuity and activity.

It is becoming increasingly more popular therefore to adopt more scientific methods of calculating staffing requirements. Two main systems are in use, both having their origins in America. These are patient dependency systems (PD) and nursing hours per patient per day systems (NHPD). Both systems allow a more specific calculation of finite staffing hours based on patient data, rather than custom and practice or subjective assessment. The merits of PD and NHPD systems to both the staffing plan and ongoing rota planning, is that, given data about occupancy and patient mix, nurse managers are able to convert this information into daily, weekly or annual nurse hours.

Patient dependency systems involve detailed timing studies of nursing activities and frequencies to establish a databank. Once the databank is set up the system functions by means of ward nurses identifying the nursing needs of individual patients on a daily basis. Figure 6.1 shows an example of the type of form used. Timings are then applied to each nursing activity to give a cumulative total of actual hours per patient. The advantage of PD systems is that they produce more accurate calculations based on patient need. Their disadvantage is that many nursing managers feel that the systems need to be computer based, which means that time and money are required to set up the database.

The NHPD system is a simpler system to calculate as it relies on average overall timings which are applied to each patient. The current range in most common use is 3.5 to 5 hours per patient day. The calculation of staffing requirements is therefore a simple calculation of number of patients multiplied by the selected average.

24 patients x 4.2 = 101 nursing hours.

Critics of the NHPD system feel that it is too crude a method of calculation in that it takes no account of patient acuity and activity and ignores the effect of day cases. I would add to that, that it also ignores the

Figure 6.1 Patient dependency classification

HOSPITAL _____ **DAY** _____
WARD/UNIT _____ **DATE** _____

	Patient Room Number											
	1	2	3	4	5	6	7	8	9	10	11	12
CARE PLANNING												
Update assess.												
Update care plan												
NURSING CARE												
COMMUNICATION												
Teaching												
Support												
DIET												
Prep. for meals												
Feed i/c help												
Total Feed												
HYGIENE												
Supervise/Instruct												
Bath i/c help												
Bath by nurse												
Oral hygiene												
ELIMINATION												
Supervise/instruct												
Toilet i/c help												
Incontinent care												
Catheter care												
MOBILITY												
Exc./Pos. in bed												
Walk i/c help												
Bedrest i/c turns												
MEDICATION												
Oral drops. Supp.												
I. M. Injection												
I.V. Injection												
Initiate I.V.I.												
Maintain I.V.I.												
Syringe Driver												
VITAL SIGNS												
Daily												
B.D.												
4 hrly												
More than 4 hrly												
VARIABLE ACTIVITIES												
Dressing Simple												
Complex												
Dr. Rounds												
Visit												
Venepuncture												
ECG												
Removal drip												
drain												
sutures												
pack												
Empty redivac												
Collect specimen												
Inhalation												
Eye care												
EVALUATION												
Evaluate care given												
Review care given												
TOTAL UNITS												
P.C. HOURS												

TOTAL HOURS _____

key factor of distribution of hours within the 24 hour period and that the derivation of the average timing which is applied to each patient is often by random selection.

A system which is a composite of the NHPD and PD system overcomes many of these criticisms, although like the PD system it involves time and cost in training nurse managers how to interpret and manage the information. This system uses average timings per patient but a range of averages is available dependent on the patient-dependency mix and admission activity. Figure 6.2 gives an example of the type of information collected.

In the current and the future climate of the health-care industry, it is clear that resource management systems such as PD and NHPD will become increasingly important. Nurse managers need this type of information for effective planning of staffing requirements and building up a historic database to use for budgeting and the staff planning process.

Effectiveness — the ability of managers to reach goals; and efficiency — the ability to reach specific goals while maintaining the predetermined allowance for cost, are key components of any managerial function. Nurse managers must therefore be prepared to invest time and commitment to resource management. Such commitment must be in a positive sense rather than the current all too common practice of justifying practices and staffing levels which have more basis in tradition than in objective reasoning.

Whatever system of resource management is used, account must again be taken by nurse managers of the internal and external factors, for their contribution towards staffing requirements. Inefficient systems, low productivity and non-nursing duties will, if unresolved, pressurise even the most rational and precise staffing calculations. Nurse managers must look behind the obvious for the reasons why staff are requesting additional nursing time. To accept such requests at face value will often lead to inappropriate decisions because the real problems remain unidentified. The most common justification for requests for additional staffing is the workload of high dependency patients and yet studies reveal that the proportion of high dependency patients in the average independent hospital is relatively low and that nurses routinely over-estimate the actual dependency of their patient workload. Nurse managers must become more objective and analytical therefore and look at all the factors affecting staffing for their contribution. Commonly it is found that it is the combination of several factors which pressurises staffing levels and not the single factor of dependency.

Calculating a staffing plan

Patient dependency and NHPD systems are valuable for calculations on which a staffing plan can be based. The staffing plan is the determination of how many nurses will be required against a predetermined occupancy. The annual budget provides the forecast occupancy figures for the year.

Figure 6.2 Composite method for staffing requirements calculation

DAILY ANALYSIS FORM

HOSPITAL _____   WARD _____

DAY _____   DATE _____

Completed by _____

No. of operational beds _____

CENSUS	AM	PM	AV.	LBR.STD.	HOURS
DAY CASES	AM	PM			HOURS
ADMISSIONS	AM		AFT.		EVE.
DISCHARGES					
DEPENDENCY	LOW		MEDIUM		HIGH
SPECIAL	CHARGED		NOT CHARGED		HOURS
THEATRE	AM		AFT.		EVE.
Minor					
Inter					
Major					
Major+					

STAFFING

	PERM.	BANK	AGENCY	GRADE			TOTAL
				RN	EN	AUX	
MORNING							
AFTERNOON							
EVENING							
NIGHT							

TOTAL HRS. ACTUAL _____ HRS. CALCULATED ____ VARIANCE _____

LABOUR STANDARD ACHIEVED _____

HOURS LOST:

Holiday _____   OPD _____

Sickness _____   Escort _____

Training _____   Admin _____

Other (please specify) _____

COMMENTS:

Using the NHPD system as an example, Fig. 6.3 shows the method of calculation for providing both an annual staffing requirement and a weekly average. Clearly the actual weekly requirement will fluctuate and therefore the staffing plan must have the flexibility to reflect these variations. The staffing plan can now take on realism through having identified the annual nursing hours required to deliver the care for budgeted occupancy.

Annual budget occupancy:-   7360 pt. days
                                   250 day case

NHPD average: I.P.   4.3 ⎫
                   D.C.   3.0 ⎬ example norms
                              ⎭

    7360 x 4.3 =   31,648 staff hours annually
    250 x 3.0 =   750 staff hours annually
                   _____

                   32,398
                   _____

    32,398/52 (weeks) = 623 hours per week
         623/37.5 = 16.6 FTE (excluding annual leave)

Figure 6.3 Calculating staffing requirement by NHPD system

The next stage in developing the staffing plan is deciding the composition of the annual staffing hours. At present three models are most commonly used for this process. The first of these is the traditional model which uses 80-90 per cent full time permanent nurses to fulfil the annual plan with some top-up by bank nursing staff. The second model, which still predominates within the independent sector, uses a combination of contract and bank staff to fulfil the annual staffing requirements. The proportion of contract to bank hours is variable but typically 60-70 per cent of the annual hours would be serviced by contract staff. The third model, which is becoming increasingly popular again uses 80-90 per cent permanent nurse hours but avoids the problems of overstaffing by use of a variety of employment contracts: 3-month fixed term, 40-week contracts and variable part time. These enable the contract hours to be altered in response to seasonal variations (see Fig. 6.4).

The effects of the three models are shown in Fig. 6.4 where the annual occupancy is broken down into monthly budgeted figures. The peaks and troughs in occupancy which are an integral part of the industry, reveal the problems of staffing plans based on Models 1 and 2. Model 1 will produce overstaffing during some months of the year which can only be ameliorated to a minor extent by annual leave. Model 2 on the other hand will

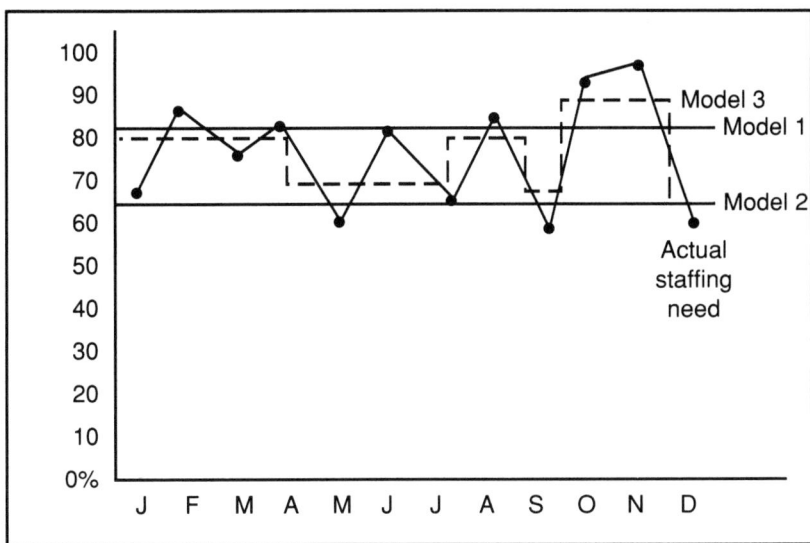

Figure 6.4 Control of contract hours by employment contracts

seldom result in overstaffing but the practical problems of providing and supervising bank nurses in the numbers required to supplement contract nurses, are becoming increasingly difficult. Model 3 attempts to overcome these problems by varying the levels of contract staff to match peaks and troughs, through the use of fixed term, school-term and 40-week contracts. The main importance is that nurse managers recognise the value of alternative staffing plans and do not treat their existing plan as fixed and unchangeable. A plan which is appropriate for the commissioning and early life of a hospital may well become less appropriate as the hospital matures and trends change.

Staffing hours

Having calculated the annual nursing hours required and the contract to bank nurse mix, the next decision for the nurse manager is the proportion of full to part-time nurses. Again, past experience and custom and practice are often evident in influencing such decisions. Part-time employees were for many years held in low regard in the NHS and their use was heavily limited and constrained. Many nurse managers may themselves have had bad experiences with poorly motivated or out-of-date part-time nurses, who were more of a burden than a bonus to the hospital. Sadly such experiences and practices have set low expectations and value in the minds of some nurse managers. Yet a far more flexible and appropriate distribution of nursing hours can be achieved through the addition of part-time nurses. Their use can strengthen the specific days of the week and parts of the day when workload is known to be heaviest and schooltime, short-term and 40-week contracts which provide flexibility to the annual staffing plan are often of interest to the part-time nurse. With the growing shortage of nurses, it is an irony that studies in recent years have identified large numbers of nurses in the community as young mothers, who do not return to work because of the inflexibility of hours and conditions of employment. Undoubtedly more accommodation of the needs of working mothers will have to be achieved in the future, as the availability of newly qualified nurses diminishes. The experience in other service industries facing similar problems demonstrates that they have achieved remarkable success in attracting employees to return to work. Job-share schemes, flexible working hours and back-to-work training are just some of the strategies which companies have employed to aid recruitment.

Staffing mix

Decisions concerning staffing mix will be influenced partly by the availability of certain grades within the local community and partly by the type and nature of the work to be undertaken. Efficiency in utilisation of personnel and quality of care delivered, are the basic criteria for determining the mix. It is important therefore to consider the exact nature of the work to be done and the most appropriate level of personnel to undertake that work. Such deliberations may well identify that a substantial amount of work is clerical or administrative in nature. It is uneconomic to incorporate this type of task routinely in the nurses' work and can often result in a poorer standard, since it is likely that the nurses' aptitude and motivation for these tasks are not very great. This also applies to other types of work such as housekeeping, catering and stores. One recent manpower study by the NHS Management Consultancy Service revealed that the average time spent on direct patient care ranged from as little as 34.4 to 56.2 per cent. Studies in the independent sector indicate similar ratios. Yet another study on nursing shortages revealed that Britain is second in the league table for the Western World in the number of nurses per occupied bed. This report concludes that if health care managers stopped using nurses for non-nursing tasks, they would be able to cope with the manpower shortages and simultaneously reduce staffing costs. Ward clerks, personal assistants and receptionists may therefore be appropriate personnel to include within the staffing mix.

As an enabling process to the effective utilisation of non-nursing personnel, nurses and managers must examine their own attitudes and perceptions. Many examples can be found of under utilisation of non-nursing staff because of the reluctance of nurses to relinquish non-nursing duties and because of their lack of confidence in the wider range of duties such personnel might be trained to undertake. No debates on staffing mix would be complete without comment on the introduction of the support worker. The first pilot schemes for Project 2000 are due to commence later this year and therefore the support worker is soon to become a reality rather than another academic debate. Many managers feel that the introduction of a new level within the nursing team will have little effect on the independent sector. However, like the nursing process, primary nursing and many other NHS initiatives, it is likely to be only a question of time before the initiative affects both sectors alike. Managers need to be considering and planning now for the eventuality that the skill mix will need to change in the future to both train and accommodate the support worker.

In addition to identifying the potential for using support personnel, the analysis of the nature of the work will help to identify the mix of nursing staff. Obviously if the nature of the work is primarily high-dependency, high-technology, then a greater proportion of sister and RGN grades will be indicated. For a broad spectrum of general work a spread of RGN and EN grades will be preferable. When making such decisions, whilst it is necessary to employ sufficient sister and RGN grades to discharge the management and supervisory functions, it must be borne in mind that a structure which is too heavy with sister and RGN grades can have a demotivating effect both on these nurses and on the nurses below them. Opportunities for job satisfaction and responsibility become dissipated and often frustration and boredom can result. Such can also be the effect of too many nurse management tiers, without any additional perceived benefit. The trend within the profession currently is to reduce the management pyramid, flattening the nursing hierarchy and delegating more authority to the ward departmental sister and her team.

Staffing rotas

Staff rotas are the final stage in the staff planning process, where nurses are assigned to specific days and hours of work. Staff rostering uses the resources designated by the staffing plan and the chief goal for effective rostering is accurately balancing staffing hours to patient workload. Clearly a PD or NHPD management system is a valuable tool in this process.

Several different patterns of rostering are in use within the profession of which the most common is a set distribution of nursing hours throughout the week and throughout the 24-hour period — 40 per cent morning, 30 per cent evening and 30 per cent night duty. (see Fig. 6.5)

Figure 6.5 maps out the peaks and troughs of workload which occur within a typical day and demonstrates how the percentage distribution method can produce understaffing and overstaffing within the 24-hour period. Newer models of rostering are overcoming this by a staggered distribution of working hours, better able to reflect workload. These models make use of the flexitime concept where instead of fixed shifts, staff hours are flexibly distributed within the day and within the week as needed. There is a crediting and debiting of hours from one week onto the next, the only mandate being that the contracted number of hours

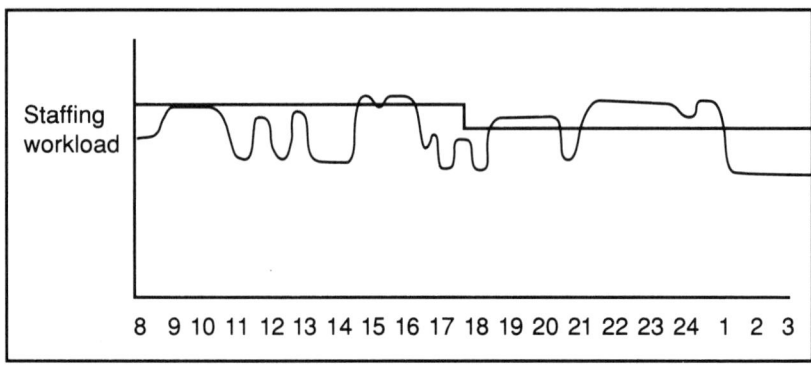

Figure 6.5 Fluctuations in staff workload

must have been worked by the end of the month. Despite initial misgivings, many hospitals trying this system are reporting its popularity with the staff, a better correlation of staff to workload and a reduction in staffing costs. It must be said, however, that consultation, flexibility and sensitivity in implementation are essential to its success.

Staff management

No discussion on staffing can be complete without at least some mention about staff management. Management styles, leadership, job content, challenge and achievement are just some of the elements that affect our motivation, commitment and productivity. Any manager knows the worth of enthusiastic and committed individuals who will outperform many others. A number of misconceptions still exist amongst managers about how best to create a productive environment. Such misconceptions have led to an over-zealous concentration on such things as terms and conditions, relationships and status. Maslow, Hertzberg and others point out quite clearly that whilst these things can demotivate, their mere presence will not of itself motivate. What does make people feel good about their work is achievement, recognition, interesting and worthwhile job, involvement and responsibility. Recent studies reveal that a great many nurses are leaving the profession not because of salary and conditions but because of the absence of these motivating factors. The contribution of the psychology of human behaviour is indeed considerable in tackling such problems. Knowing how to get the best out of people, how to create the conditions in which they will perform to their best and applying this knowledge to the work environment is crucial to effective management. Good resource management will serve to get the right people, in the right place at the right time. It takes good staff management then to ensure that they perform to their full capacity and optimum standard.

References

Out of Touch with Patients? NHS Management Services 1989 *Nursing Times* April

Nursing a Grievance 1987 *The Economist* August

7 Registration and inspection
Paul Ridout

The independent sector welcomes rules that help set a high standard for private hospitals and homes. There has however been much concern at the way in which these rules are applied, and a feeling that Health Authorities are sometimes setting higher standards for the private sector than they themselves can achieve. We asked a lawyer to write this chapter because the legislation is of some complexity.

Introduction

In this chapter I shall attempt to describe the procedure and institutions concerned in the registration of nursing homes in England and Wales. This legislation covers both 'private hospitals' and 'nursing homes', but refers to them as 'nursing homes' throughout. Different rules apply in Scotland, Northern Ireland, the Isle of Man and the Channel Islands. The aim is to provide the reader with an overview of the registration process of nursing homes. This chapter does not deal with the registration of residential care homes where rules, procedures and practices, although similar, have some significant differences.

History

The forerunner of the modern law relating to the registration of nursing homes was Section 187 of the Public Health Act 1936 which provided for a simple procedure of registration of nursing homes with the local county council. By 1975 the profile of the industry had increased to such an extent that Parliament decided to place the rules relating to a nursing home registration in one Act, the Nursing Homes Act 1975 and although this introduced some changes it was in essence an Act of consolidation.

A similar process led to the Registered Homes Act 1984, the statute which currently governs this subject.

The Registered Homes Act 1984 has acquired a completely undeserved reputation as a watershed in the law relating to nursing home registration. The watershed I would suggest was recognition by Government (both central and local) that the nursing home industry had grown into a substantial provider of medical services to significant numbers of members of the public and had ceased to be a fringe operation ancillary to the practice of medicine and nursing. No doubt this was caused in part by a political atmosphere providing a warmer climate for private medical practice but, I suggest, by far the greatest influence was the decision by Government in the early 1980s to provide limitless cash to pay for the true cost of accommodation and nursing for those in need of nursing care in private establishments. The boom created by that decision in the 1980s was abruptly stopped by an equally arbitrary decision of Government to limit such cash spending from April 1985. We may well see that the next piece of legislation to be introduced in the field of nursing-home registration owes its birth to that decision. Social Security benefits for nursing home patients are dealt with in annex to Chapter 3.

Despite its reputation the Registered Homes Act 1984 did no more than consolidate the existing legislation, combine rules for nursing homes and the rules for Residential Care Homes into one Act and, most importantly, create the new appeal procedure of the Registered Homes Tribunal.

One often hears those concerned with the implementation of nursing home registration practice speak of the change effected in 1984. The change was one of recognition of an industry by Government rather than a dramatic change in the rules and that point is an important argument in debates which centre upon an assertion that standards of other matters changed with the Registered Homes Act 1984.

Source material

There are certain essential items of source material necessary to consider a problem relating to Nursing Home registration. I shall group these in two sections and give to each a short title for future use in this chapter.

Section A

1 Registered Homes Act 1984 (the 1984 Act).

2 The Nursing Homes and Mental Nursing Homes Regulations 1984 (the 1984 Regulations).

3 The Registered Homes Tribunals Rules 1984 (the RHT Rules).

4 The Nursing Homes and Mental Nursing Homes (Amendment) Regulations 1986 (the 1986 Regulations). The Nursing Homes and Mental

Nursing Homes (Amendment) Regulations 1988 (the 1988 Regulations).

5 The Directive by The Secretary of State dated September 1984 (the 1984 Directive).

   NB: This is to be found at Annex C to the *National Association of Health Authorities Hand Book on Registration and Inspection of Nursing Homes.*

6 A *Handbook for Health Authorities upon the Registration and Inspection of Nursing Homes* issued by the National Association of Health Authorities in 1985 (together 'the NAHA Guidelines').

7 The 1988 Supplement to the NAHA Guidelines.

I would urge everyone concerned on a day-to-day basis with registration or operation of nursing homes to have a copy of each item listed above readily available.

Section B

1 The National Health Service Act 1977 (the 1977 Act).

2 The National Health Service Functions (Directions to Authorities and Administration Arrangements) Regulations 1989 (the NHS 1989 Regulations) [replaces the 1982 Regulations].

3 The Nurses Midwives and Health Visitors Act 1979 (the 1979 Nurses Act).

4 The Nurses Midwives and Health Visitors Rules Approval Order 1983 (the Nurses Rules 1983).

5 The Nurses Midwives and Health Visitors (Parts of the Register) Order 1983 (the Nurses Register Order).

6 A complete set of the reported Decisions of Registered Homes Tribunals.

This additional source material will be of vital use to those more particularly concerned with individual legal problems and it would certainly be a useful addition to the office library of a nurse manager or a health authority registration officer.

What is a nursing home?

A nursing home is a legal term exclusively defined in Section 21 of the 1984 Act. A mental nursing home is defined in Section 22 of the 1984 Act.

   For any particular case the student or adviser must study the sections very carefully. However it may be broadly stated that a nursing home encompasses a very much wider group of buildings and institutions than are included in the popular conception of the term 'nursing home'.

In the broadest terms nursing homes are places for the care of the sick, the injured and the infirm.

Surprisingly this will extend to any centres for the provision of medical care unless excluded by the 1984 Act.

Hospitals are excluded only if operated by Government central or local, or by bodies instituted by special Act of Parliament or Royal Charter.

Premises providing medical attention ancillary to the main purpose of buildings in which they are placed, e.g. at school or in workplace will be excluded. Private dwellings are excluded as are the surgeries of doctors, dentists and chiropodists.

However if premises are not excluded and if the premises are used to provide nursing care they must be registered. To provide nursing care in premises not registered (or otherwise under lawful permission, e.g. in NHS hospitals) is a criminal offence.

There are and will continue to be anomalies.

An institution providing nursing care and education to the chronically sick young may require registration both as a nursing home and as a school.

Day centres which provide nursing care require registration. This should be contrasted with day centres with provision of personal and/or social care which do not require registration.

Curiously, the exclusion of a private dwelling is not limited to the private dwelling of the person receiving the nursing service. Therefore a domiciliary nursing service in the patient's home does not require registration under the 1984 Act but may require registration under the Nurses Agencies Act or the Employment Agencies Act 1973. An individual who uses his private house to a limited extent to provide nursing care on a day or residential basis seems not to require to register provided that he is able to show that the quality of the building has not changed from a private dwelling.

Similar problems may arise with a mental nursing home.

It is not common practice to register general nursing homes as mental nursing homes but the Act provides that a mental nursing home means premises used for the provision of nursing and medical treatment for at least one mentally disordered patient. Grave difficulties could arise in practice in differentiating between the need to register specifically as a mental nursing home or in considering whether general nursing home registration is sufficient to care for patients suffering from varying degrees of confusion and/or dementia. The problems will be exacerbated as the symptoms of the particular conditions vary on a day-to-day basis. The matter is further confused by the section of the Act dealing with registration of residential care homes which provides that premises must be registered if they provide personal care for persons in need thereof *inter alia* by reason of present mental disorder. The confusion created by this multitude of statutory provisions will need to be carefully considered by anyone considering operating premises for the mentally disordered.

The persons concerned in registration

The Secretary of State for Health

Powers relating to the registration of nursing homes have been delegated by Parliament to the Secretary of State for Health. The minister is the ultimate source of power both to make regulations concerning the operation of nursing homes and to control day-to-day procedures.

The Regional Health Authority

By Sections 13 and 14 of the 1977 Act the Secretary of State is required to delegate certain of his powers including his powers in relation to nursing homes to regional health authorities (RHAs) whom in turn he must require to sub-delegate those powers to district health authorities (DHAs).

The delegation was achieved by the NHS 1982 Regulations and revised by the NHS 1984 Amendment Regulations simply to take into account the changes of statutory reference between the Nursing Homes Act 1975 and the 1984 Act.

It is, however, vital to note that the Secretary of State has reserved to himself regulation-making power. Therefore neither RHAs nor DHAs have power to make regulations binding in law in relation to Nursing Homes.

District Health Authorities

Power delegated by the Secretary of State to RHAs has been compulsorily subdelegated to DHAs but there should be an instrument of delegation to which reference should be made in appropriate cases. The source of the DHA power is its instrument of subdelegation from the RHA who have acquired their power from the Secretary of State. Any limitations in that subdelegation may affect the power of the DHA to operate in a particular case and both health authority administrators and those advising nursing home proprietors in appropriate cases should consult that documentation.

It is the DHA as a body which is required to take decisions in relation to registration, variation of registration and where appropriate cancellation of registration. A DHA would be unwise to subdelegate its powers to nominated officers as it can be argued that those officers have no delegated power to make decisions of their own accord but are merely servants of the Authority. Therefore a certificate of registration issued by an officer or a proposal to cancel a registration signed by an officer without the authority of a resolution of the DHA may very well be found invalid. Officers and members of DHAs contemplating action under the 1984 Act should bear this in mind and not expose themselves to the risk of technical points being taken against them by nursing home proprietors and their advisers.

In addition the DHA is empowered and indeed obliged (see the 1984 Directive) to inspect all nursing homes within its area *and* all premises which it has reasonable cause to believe are being used for nursing purposes. This power and duty of inspection may be subdelegated (see Regulation 10 of the 1984 Regulations) and this brings us to the health authority officer.

Health authority officer

The health authority officer will be an employee of the health authority specifically engaged to deal with nursing home registration problems. In relation to applications for registration or the consideration of proposals for cancellation of registration this officer is the complete servant of the authority and in performing his duty is carrying out the wishes of the authority. He is not acting on his own account. Unfortunately many DHAs rubber stamp the decisions of their officers. It is suggested that that is wrong. The health authority is thereby avoiding the duty given by Parliament. Problems would be avoided if health authorities were to consider the recommendations of their officers on an equal footing with those of the private nursing home owner. A nursing home officer, however, has power if properly authorised, to inspect nursing homes. Thus if authorised by a proper document this officer may require entry to a nursing home at any time of the day or night and he may not be refused entry. However his power is limited to inspect and to report back, and it is not a power to direct nursing home proprietors as to how they should run their businesses.

The person in charge

The person in charge of a nursing home is the person responsible for the professional nursing case of the patients accommodated in the nursing home. That person may or may not be a proprietor of the nursing home. The DHA does not have the power to veto a particular appointment but it must be advised of the identity of the person in charge and of his or her qualifications. Subject to that, the appointment of a person in charge is a matter for the nursing home proprietor who should not allow himself to be inhibited in making his own employment choice by any form of apparent over-influence from the DHA. This has the power to propose cancellation of registration if it is satisfied (and a heavy burden of proof is required) that by reason of the identity of the person in charge the home is not fit to operate as a nursing home. It will be noted that it is simply the failure to provide an appropriately qualified person to be person in charge which is the ground for registration refusal or cancellation not the quality, professional experience or other personal attributes of the person selected.

Health authorities would be well advised to consider the gravity of suggesting that a professional doctor or nurse is not fit to carry out the task for which they are professionally qualified.

The 1984 Directive provides that the person in charge must be, if a nurse, a nurse registered as a first level nurse in the 1979 Nurses Act extended by the Nurses Register Order.

The home owner

The home owner is the most important person concerned in the operation of a nursing home. It is his or her own business. It is for the home owner to decide how the business should be operated, advised and persuaded by other professionals where appropriate, but not intimidated or coerced into a course of action by the registration authority. Registration officers are not entitled to dictate the manner of operation of a home or the style in which the home shall be equipped or furnished. Only if the home's standard of adequacy is such or reaches such a point that by reason of some factor or other it may be shown on the balance of probabilities that the home is unfit for use as a nursing home does the DHA have powers to intervene. Matters of taste and individual modes of operation are for the home owner. The corollary is that if things go wrong it will be the home owner who legally takes the blame and he will not be able to rely as a defence upon the premise that he was following instructions from the DHA. If, as may be the case those instructions were misconceived, it is the home owner's default. He should have taken the right course.

The Certificate of Registration

The Certificate of Registration is the documentary evidence signifying that the particular proprietor is entitled to carry on the nursing home business subject to certain conditions. It is unlawful to carry on a nursing home without a Certificate or in contravention of the conditions. This is an absolute rule and breach is a criminal offence. No matter how strong the morality (as seen by the home owner) of the particularly persuasive circumstance of the case, the first and principal rule of nursing home law is that there must be a Certificate and the valid conditions on the Certificate must be obeyed.

No nursing home proprietor should commence in business until the Certificate has been obtained. This does create difficulty. The corollary is that no health authority should issue a Certificate until it is satisfied that the home is ready to operate. The Certificate is a licence to operate a nursing home. In practical terms many DHAs issue Certificates subject to undertakings for further work and subject to undertakings as to the employment of staff. Clearly a working arrangement is very helpful but if a DHA entertains fears it is quite justified in withholding a Certificate until it is satisfied that all essential matters have been fulfilled, before commercial operations begin. This includes complete commissioning of the home and complete engagement of the necessary staff to provide care for the number of patients for whom registration is to be granted.

Every applicant for a nursing home registration must bear this in mind. If they wish their application to be processed they must make sure that the DHA rapidly receives the information necessary to enable it to grant the application.

The Certificate of Registration is timeless. Although an annual fee is payable the annual fee is payable to assist discharge of the administrative expenses of the DHA. It is not a question of registration being reviewed upon an annual basis. The Registration Certificate is thus a valuable document. Once obtained it cannot be removed whilst the same registered owner remains proprietor of nursing home, unless the cancellation procedure is followed.

The Registration Certificate may be subject to conditions.

The High Court has decided that the only conditions which may be imposed upon a Certificate of Registration (whether by the registration authority or by the Registered Homes Tribunal on appeal) are those conditions set out in the 1984 Act. There are four such conditions.

Number of persons to be accommodated, excluding staff and relatives

It should be noted that the condition relates to persons accommodated and not patients accommodated so that if there are others within the registered premises who are not patients of the nursing home, e.g. up to three residents receiving personal care, it is arguable that the DHA can limit those numbers as well as the number of patients.

Categories of patient

The DHA can limit the category of patient who may receive care in the particular home. In an application for registration the applicant must specify the categories for whom he or she wishes to provide care and accommodation. Great difficulties can arise from overdetailed classification and categorisation of patient. Detailed categories mean that patients falling outside the detailed interpretation of the category are not lawfully receiving care. This may affect their right to receive benefit and may certainly cause the proprietors to risk being prosecuted. It is suggested that applicants should specify the broadest categories of patient to whom they propose to provide care perhaps delimited only by age. No one can foresee exactly which patients may come to a nursing home and the nursing home proprietor should not be artificially limited in the reception of patients unless it can be clearly demonstrated that a mix of certain categories would be detrimental to either category, or both. An example would be that young cancer patients or young physically disabled patients in need of nursing care might be thought not to mix satisfactorily with the elderly sick. For similar reasons it is often thought that children should only be accommodated in specialist nursing homes. Within those broad categories the majority of DHAs register simply for a maximum number of patients.

The attractions of registering to meet categories prescribed for income support purposes should be resisted as those artificial rules can be changed as easily as they are created and it is now clearly established that registration categories are not, in the case of nursing homes, a pre-condition to the patient obtaining a particular level of support.

It also seems right that in the context of specifying categories of patient it should be possible to specify areas of the nursing home suitable for limited categories of patient. The obvious categories are those who have limited mobility and those who may wander because of confusion. Such patients may need to be accommodated in areas where they are more easily overseen or where they may more easily be moved from one part of the home to another either in emergency or for the purposes of everyday living. It is suggested that it would be wrong to refuse to register a particular part of a nursing home on the ground that it was not suitable for the mostly highly dependent patient but rather that that part could be registered with a limitation on the category of patient to be accommodated there. Not all elderly patients are unable to walk up and down stairs and not all fire authorities feel that it is helpful to have patients moved up and down between levels of buildings during an emergency. Many fire authorities feel that it is better for patients to remain where they are so that they can be more easily traced in the event of a fire. Constructive and creative negotiation can provide opportunities for maximising nursing home accommodation.

Other conditions

Other conditions may be made by regulation of the Secretary of State. At the time of writing no such conditions had been made.

The minimum number of nurses

A DHA may refuse an application for registration or decide to cancel an existing registration if it is satisfied that a condition imposed by it that the number of nurses possessing such qualifications as may be specified shall be on duty in the particular home at times specified is not or will not be fulfilled (Section 25 1G and Section 25 3 of the 1984 Act). There are a number of differing interpretations about this provision.

The majority view is that this is a condition of registration and thus if it is to be imposed it must be imposed in accordance with the procedures of the 1984 Act and accordingly is subject not only to the representational objections which a proprietor may make to the DHA if dissatisfied with a proposal under Section 32 of the 1984 Act but also to appeal to a Registered Homes Tribunal.

The ability to impose conditions which affect the operation of the home is exhaustively covered in the 1984 Act and is to be construed restrictively in accordance with the High Court ruling in Warwickshire County Council v. McSweeney.

Therefore if a condition relating to staffing (or any condition) is to be imposed or varied the DHA must ensure that it follows the correct procedure and that having followed the procedure the Notice is served as a Notice carrying appropriate warnings and information as to the right of appeal and that it contains relevant material. It will be binding only in respect of relevant material.

There are two views as to what may be contained in the Notice and the argument centres upon the definition of 'nurses'.

One view is that a nurse describes a person of professional qualification and the very use of the word nurse thus means a professionally qualified nurse. Those supporting that view point to the words which follow 'nurses' namely 'possessing such qualifications' and say that if Parliament had intended to include nurses who had no qualifications it would have so legislated. They will also be able to point to the lack of any equivalent provision in relation to a residential care home where nurses are not a requirement of the staffing complement and many would suggest should not be on duty in a nursing capacity.

Supporters of this contention will also point to the 1979 Nurses Act and draw attention to those provisions which make it an offence to hold oneself out as a nurse possessing particular qualifications. This is not as strong as the former provisions of the Nurses Act 1957 which made it a criminal offence to use the word nurse about someone who was not qualified as such.

Those who contend for the contrary argue that Parliament clearly intended to limit the staff engaged in direct patient care and that the expression 'nurses' includes all such persons and may by an open interpretation of the section include those who do not have any qualifications.

It is suggested that the former proposition is to be preferred and that nurses should only include those who are professionally qualified as such.

The DHA is not without weapons against an owner who provides inadequate staff of an unqualified nature for they may either consider proposing a cancellation of the registration if the staffing is such as to lead to the conclusion that the home is unfit to continue as a nursing home or if they form the view that the direct care staff are inadequate they may serve notice to that effect upon the home owner under the 1984 Regulations and if the matter is not put to rights within a period specified in the notice then the home owner will risk prosecution before the local Magistrates Court.

It is suggested that DHAs should accept the more limited ambit of the contents of a Notice to be served under Section 25 (iii) but note upon the Notice, by way of caveat, the DHAs view as to the minimum level of care staff to be engaged to provide an adequate service. The home owner would then have clear notice of what was expected and an opportunity for challenge and if subsequently criticised to the point of proposed cancellation or prosecution would have little cause for complaint if no protest had been registered.

The strongest comfort is that it is the home owner who is responsible for providing adequate facilities and services, adequate accommodation and adequate staff. The onus lies upon the home owner to fulfil the duty and not the health authority.

The subsection does not actually state that the number of nurses to be specified shall be a minimum number of nurses but this seems the natural conclusion because the scheme of the Act makes the home owner responsible for providing adequate staffing and that, presumably, will vary on a daily or weekly basis dependent upon the particular needs of the particular patients as those fluctuate.

Applications to the District Health Authority

All applications will be made by prospective or actual home owners.

An application may either be to register a new home or to change the ownership of an existing home. The current fees upon application for a new home are £600 and the current fee upon re-registration upon change of ownership is £550.

In addition an annual fee is payable within one month after registration. This is related to the number of beds for which registration has been granted. The current rate is £22 per bed. Another annual fee will be paid upon the anniversary of payment of the first annual fee and so forth for the duration of the Licence. The current fee scale is set out in the 1988 Regulations. The information which is required of an applicant for registration or indeed an applicant for re-registration on change of ownership is set out in Schedule 2 to the 1984 Regulations. In most cases the DHA will provide a standard form. Provided that all the information required in Schedule 2 has been provided the application is a competent application but the DHA may, and indeed probably should, ask further searching questions of applicants.

Any applicant should study Schedule 2 to the 1984 Regulations carefully and there it will be seen that a DHA can if it so wishes insist that all facilities are in place before the application is granted.

It would seem sensible for DHAs to pay particular care to applications. It is very much more satisfactory to refuse an application after proper investigations than it is to find that an application has been granted in haste and then for the authority to be faced with the unpleasant time-consuming and expensive task of seeking to cancel the registration.

The DHA officer should remember that applications under the 1984 Act and 1984 Regulations are exempt from the provision of the Rehabilitation of Offenders Act 1974 so that applicants may and should be required to provide details of any previous convictions.

In this regard the standard application form which has been circulated to many authorities is significantly defective. It appears to require details of convictions imposed upon anyone to be employed in the home. This has led to confusion and has been described by a Registered Homes Tribunal as ambiguous and confusing. Clearly a DHA will be particularly concerned with the criminal records of those who are to be involved in direct patient care or direct patient contact but it is submitted that they may be equally concerned with the records of those concerned in the management and administration of a company who may have nothing to do with patients. The drafting of the form leaves open the excuse for incomplete preparation that the applicants had not appreciated that information should be supplied in connection with all those connected with the proposed operation.

Financial capabilities of applicants

It is suggested, although this may be controversial, that DHAs would be well advised to enquire in depth into the financial capabilities of the applicants. The authority needs to know that financial resources are adequate to meet the running costs of the home without any risk of temporary suspension. The authority needs to know that the home is able to meet its financial charges, its staff costs and its overheads easily within the income generated. A small home with low finance may operate perfectly satisfactorily. If a purchaser increases the amount of the borrowing secured against the home and repayable out of the earnings so as to facilitate the purchase the whole viability of the home may change.

It also seems advisable for DHAs to enquire into the motives and reasons why the particular applicant has decided to venture into the nursing home business.

The authority will be determining whether or not the applicant is a fit person to carry on the business of a nursing home and it is suggested to DHAs and indeed to applicants that they may only discharge their function with searching enquiries.

Applications for registration are time-consuming and will have to compete for the time of the relevant DHA officers with other duties. If the DHA has ordered its affairs correctly it will, it is suggested, leave the decision upon an application to a meeting of the authority or maybe to a specified subcommittee of the authority who will report back. Both a subcommittee and the authority itself will pay particular attention to the advice that it received from its officers. A prudent applicant should acquaint him or herself with the timescale for considering applications. Nothing is more frustrating than a delayed application but experience shows that the vast majority of delayed applications are caused not by obstructive behaviour on the part of the DHA officers or members but because applicants have simply not provided the appropriate information in time for the officers to make a recommendation. By way of example the commissioning of the home must be completed in sufficient time before the appropriate meeting of the DHA to enable the officers to inspect and report back.

Conditional approval

The problems that arise because applicants are unwilling to commit themselves to substantial capital expenditure or the engagement of staff who will be paid without work or may have become disaffected whilst waiting for work to start can, it is suggested, be overcome on a case-by-case basis by the provisions being agreed between the officers and the applicant subject to ratification by the authority, the applicants giving an appropriately detailed undertaking and in reliance upon that undertaking the authority either issuing the Certificate with instructions to its officers not to date and release it until they are satisfied that the undertakings are fulfilled or in a particular case (and certainly not generally) instructing a particular member, perhaps the chairman of the Health Authority, or an officer to sign the Certificate once and only once satisfied that the undertakings have been fulfilled.

It is convenient to mention another serious defect in the standard form of application. This incorporates an undertaking immediately above the signature clause that the applicants will abide by the provisions of what is described as the Guide to Registration. As far as is known no such document exists. It is possible that the term might refer to individual guidelines for registration issued by authorities from time to time and district by district. That it is suggested would be a thoroughly bad practice. If it were to be asserted that the applicant by having signed such an application form became bound by the rigid terms of guidelines which were not otherwise enforceable by law, the position would be less than satisfactory. All applicants faced with such a form are recommended to delete the appropriate provisions. Neither the 1984 Regulations nor the 1984 Act require signature of such a declaration. It is possible in an extreme case, where there was a dispute upon the standards found in a home that a Magistrates Court or a Registered Homes Tribunal might find a proprietor bound by the terms of the guidelines if he had signed such a form when they would not regard him as so bound if there were no such declaration.

Variation application

Once registered a home owner may wish to vary conditions of registration by changing the categories of patients for whom care may be provided or in most cases by increasing the numbers for whom care may be provided. The most obvious example is a building extension to a nursing home which has become successfully established so as to increase profitability. Surprisingly there is no direct statutory authority for an application to vary conditions. Regulation 6 of the 1984 Regulations provides that the DHA may vary conditions. The standard practice adopted is that applications are accepted from home owners for the variation of registration conditions as if they were applications for registration. As a matter of practice DHAs take an individual view about such applications in determining whether or not applications are so extensive as to be a brand new application or whether the application is of a minor nature so that it may be treated as a simple variation application attracting a lower fee. A brand new application will attract the full fees. A variation application may attract no fee if it simply relates to categories or staffing conditions or, if it relates to numbers for whom accommodation may be provided, will attract an additional annual fee as and when granted.

Section 31 of the 1984 Act provides a procedure for variation applications.

The DHA must make a written proposal as to the manner in which it proposes to vary a condition and must give notice to the home owner of the right to make representations about the variation.

Those representations may be made orally or in writing and notification of the desire to make representations must be made within fourteen days from the date of the service of proposal. The fourteen days relate not to the making of the representations but to the giving of a Notice of Intention so as to make representations. The representations themselves whether orally or in writing must be made within a reasonable time. The DHA may not make a final decision until either the representations have been heard or a reasonable time has elapsed and no representations have been made.

The representations having been heard or none having been made then the DHA may proceed to make the decision. That decision is subject to appeal to the Registered Homes Tribunal. Notice of the right of appeal must be endorsed on the written decision. That appeal may be made to a Registered Home Tribunal within twenty-eight days of service of the decision of the DHA upon the home owner.

There appears to be no provision for extending the time for delivery of Notice of Appeal (which is a simple process) and it is then submitted that otherwise than by agreement there is no room for application to extend the time for appeal or for the High Court to grant an extension.

It is crucial that those advising respective appellants know of the time limit and observe it. The Notice of Appeal is a simple statement of intention to appeal. No complicated grounds or evidence need to be prepared at that stage.

Regulation 6 of the 1984 Regulations appears to suggest that a Notice varying conditions may be served upon the home owner specifying a date upon which it shall take effect, which date shall be reasonable. This appears to be in conflict with Sections 31-34 of the 1984 Act. It is suggested that Regulation 6 cannot possibly override the effect of primary legislation and that the DHA cannot vary conditions unless they follow the procedures set out in the 1984 Act and that to this extent Regulation 6 was drafted inadvisedly and is not of effect.

Finally, applicants or those dissatisfied with decisions or prospective decisions of DHAs should read carefully Section 23 (4) of the 1984 Act. The subsection appears to suggest that the DHA must grant a certificate or by analogy the application for variation. That view found favour with the High Court in Warwickshire County Council v. McSweeney, Mr Justice Roch ruled that Registration Authorities (he was dealing with residential care homes but the same principles clearly apply to nursing homes) are under a duty to register and may only refuse if they are satisfied that grounds for refusal exist and that those grounds for refusal must be interpreted restrictively.

It is clearly established that it is for the DHA to establish and justify the grounds for its decision. The burden of proof at a Registered Homes

Tribunal will lie upon the authority which will always be respondent to the appeal and will always have to justify its decision. The DHA will have to prove its reason for rejecting the particular application or making the particular decision to cancel as justified on the balance of probabilities.

An application to a DHA must be clearly distinguished from other applications made to other local authorities e.g. a planning application. In applications such as planning applications it is clear that the authority has a wide-ranging discretion to make a decision on policy grounds. It is suggested that such a facility is not granted to a DHA considering a nursing home application. The authority is a part of an application and appeal procedure. The authority is not entitled to make policies as to the manner in which nursing homes shall operate within its jurisdiction. The authority is not just subject to appeal if it errs on points of law but it is subject to appeal to a Tribunal who will reconsider and possibly overrule its decision on the merits.

Applicants to DHAs should be aware of this restricted power on the part of the authority and not be discouraged from pressing applications which appear at first blush to be received unfavourably by officers or particular members of DHAs for whatever reason. DHA members, officers and managers should bear in mind at all stages of such applications that applications do not fall to be determined by reference to their own individual local policies but once made are subject to review in the Registered Home Tribunal and the presentation of such an appeal will be expensive of time and money and may provide public embarrassment to an authority if its decision is overturned and shown to have been made idly or without proper consideration of all the circumstances or in a perverse manner. It is felt at the present time that both members and officers of DHAs have not fully appreciated the limitations on their powers to intervene in such matters.

Operation and administration

Once he has achieved registration of his nursing home the proprietor is responsible for operating it in accordance with proper standards and proper practices. The statutory code does not delimit in a detailed way the manner in which a home is to be operated.

The rules are set out in the 1984 Regulations. These Regulations succeed in identical terms former Regulations of 1981 and have not been the subject of subsequent amendment save that the fees payable to the registration authority have been increased from time to time.

Regulations provide four areas in which a home owner is required to restrict the manner in which the home is operated. These are considered in the following sections.

Regulation 7

Regulation 7 provides certain minimum records which the home owner should keep. Home owners should note that good practice and other legal provisions may require or indicate the keeping of other records. The records specified in Regulation 7 are mandatory, they are as follows:-

- A register of patients including the information in Schedule 4.
- A register of surgical operations and the use of special techniques.
- A record of the patients' health and condition, of treatment given upon a daily basis.
- A record of all staff employed at the home.
- A record of all fire practices and fire alarm tests and procedures to be followed in the event of fire.
- A maintenance record on all medical surgical and nursing equipment.

All these records must be kept and should be available upon inspection.

Examples of other records which should be kept are records of employment history which will be important to judge employment decisions in relation to staff and may be important if there are disputes with staff.

With regard to patients, good nursing practice now dictates that a care plan should be prepared and updated in respect of each patient and this will in most cases go further than a simple statement of the patient's health and condition and the treatment provided. The nurse or doctor in charge should positively plan the care and regularly review the plan.

There is no statutory requirement for a care plan but it is suggested that absence of a care plan would reflect adversely upon the professional staff and might arouse suspicions as to the adequacy of care provided.

Deaths

The person registered must give notice of a death to the DHA within twenty-four hours of that death. There are exceptions for Bank Holiday periods extending the time.

Absence of person in charge

The DHA is entitled to receive notice of the absence of the person in charge if that person is to be away for more than four weeks. The notice should be given at least one month before the absence unless a shorter period is agreed and if there is an emergency not later than one week after the start of the absence.

Upon return the person in charge or the person registered shall notify the return to the DHA.

Some DHAs have suggested that they are entitled to receive notice if there is an absence for a shorter period. That is not so. Home owners when planning holiday arrangements for the person in charge would do well to bear in mind that shorter absence than twenty-eight days does not require a notice. It may be thought prudent to avoid the necessity to give a notice as knowledge of the absence of the person in charge may lead to unnecessary concern from the DHA which may in itself prove disrupting to the operation of the home. In any event it is suggested that continuous twenty-eight-day absence from duty is barely consistent with accepting the role of the person in charge of a large number of sick patients.

Standard of adequacy

Regulation 12 of the 1984 Regulations sets out standards for facilities and services to be provided at the home. It is not proposed to list them here. However the standard to be applied is universally described as one of adequacy. Adequacy is clearly an objective test. Thus the standard for any facility or service will be judged objectively taking into account the particular home, the category of patient and the needs of the patient.

What is or is not adequate will ultimately be judged by an outsider with a suitable amount of professional knowledge as to the operation of nursing homes. What can be stated categorically is that the standard is neither set by the authority or by its officers whether by personal decision or by the institution of guidelines, rules or policies nor is it set at the sole discretion of the home owner. Home owners are warned that they must accept constructive criticism of the standards in their home provided that criticism can be justified by reference to academic opinion and professional practice and health authorities are warned that it is beyond their power to seek to dictate or set precise delimitations of standards as to facilities or services.

The home owner must be aware that failure to provide adequate services is an offence under the Regulations. However there is some protection, for no prosecution may be brought (except in cases where the DHA is seeking or has obtained an Emergency Closure Order under Section 30 of the 1984 Act unless DHAs shall have served upon the home owner a Notice specifying the provisions in the Regulations in respect of which a failure is alleged in the Authority's opinion, the action which is required together with the period in which the action should be taken).

It is to be noted that failure to take action to comply with the authority's opinion is not an offence. It is failure to provide adequate service or facility which is the offence. The purpose of the Notice is to give the home owner warning of what is the health authority's opinion and an opportunity, if the owner is minded to accept that opinion, to put matters right without the need for prosecution.

A home owner who disagreed, after proper considerations and proper professional consultation, with the opinions expressed in a Notice should not ignore it or be constrained by the fear of prosecution to take action which he genuinely believes is inappropriate but rather should set forth in writing his objections and reasons supported where appropriate by the professional opinions relevant to the matter and indicate to the authority that the opinion is not accepted and accordingly the action will not be taken.

Home owners are warned that a positive case of disagreement with the authority is not likely to be well received before the magistrates if the case emerges for the first time in front of the magistrates. A person who has a sensible case to put forward in opposition to the DHA officer's opinion will want to make that case at the first available opportunity.

Nevertheless, in terms of a criminal offence DHAs are reminded that to succeed upon a prosecution they will have to prove the inadequacy of the service or facility beyond all reasonable doubt. The service of the Notice is a precondition to prosecution; it does not, it is submitted, switch the burden of proof onto the home owner.

It seems to the writer that, save in the most obvious of cases, the proposition that a particular service or facility can be proven inadequate beyond all reasonable doubt is a very difficult one to establish, indeed almost impossible to establish if there is sensible professional opinion taking a view which opposes the prosecutor.

It is submitted that it would be wrong in practice to use the prosecution procedure to seek to establish minimum standards of adequacy. A failure in prosecution does not establish that a particular service or facility was adequate, merely that its inadequacy was not proved beyond all reasonable doubt. It is suggested that this criminal sanction procedure should only be used in the most obvious cases where there is no professional dispute as to the particular standards of care in question.

Guidelines

This section is a convenient place to discuss the question of guidelines for the registration and inspection of nursing homes. When the 1984 Act was passed the DHSS recommended to all DHAs that they should prepare guidelines for nursing home owners, their own officers and prospective nursing home owners as to the registration and inspection procedure. Most DHAs have issued such guidelines and guidelines have been issued by the National Association of Health Authorities in their Handbook of 1985 supplemented in 1988.

Decisions of Registered Homes Tribunals have unanimously supported the original proposition that the guidelines were nothing more than guidance. They are not rules of law and they are not irrefutable. As a matter of practice the NAHA Guidelines will be regarded with great respect by Registered Homes Tribunals or others in a responsible position in the nursing home industry. In assessing the adequacy or otherwise of particular standards any deviation from the norms established in the NAHA Guidelines will come under critical review. Thus health authorities who seek to impose standards above and beyond those recommended by NAHA will find themselves in grave difficulties in holding these standards either before the Magistrates Court or in the Registered Homes Tribunal. Conversely the home owner who seeks to justify standards which fall below those set out in the NAHA Guidelines will find himself struggling. Every case is determined on its own merits and there may be exceptions. In one case a Registered Homes Tribunal held that a room was sufficient to accommodate two people because of its peculiarly attractive situation and the particular position of the home and the category of residents there. That room not only fell short in size of the particular DHA minimum guidelines but also fell below the minimum recommended size in the NAHA Guidelines which were significantly different from the DHA guidelines.

Great caution should be exercised before seeking to establish or justify a practice, procedure, service or facility which is not at least at the minimum level recommended by NAHA.

Inspection of nursing homes

The DHA is entitled to inspect any premises carried on as a nursing home at any time of the day or night without prior appointment.

By the 1984 Directive a DHA is obliged to inspect any premises within its area which it has reasonable cause to believe are being used as a nursing home.

A DHA is obliged to inspect every nursing home within its area not less frequently than twice every twelve months.

The difference between premises registered as a nursing home and premises not so registered is that in the former case the DHA representative is entitled as of right to inspect but in the case of other premises the DHA representative must have reasonable cause to believe that he will discover activities which may be proved to be provision of nursing care within the premises.

DHA officers must remember that unless they are able to say that they have evidence (which can be proved at a later date) that the premises are used for nursing purposes they have no right to enter and may be refused entry. The corollary is that if entry is forced and there were no reasonable grounds to suspect the commission of an offence then the entry is unlawful, amounts to trespass to land and may involve the individual officer and the DHA in a claim for damages.

It matters not whether or not the practice of nursing is discovered on inspection, what is important is that the authority must have had reasonable cause to suspect that they might discover such activities.

DHA officers will remember that it is not an offence to carry on nursing within a private dwelling house provided that the private dwelling house has not been so adapted that its main purpose is seen to be the provision of nursing.

DHA officers should also remember that notwithstanding that a resident in a residential care home may be considered to be in need of nursing care, premises would only require registration as a nursing home with their local authority if nursing care is being provided. Probably the failure to provide nursing care to a resident in need could amount to an offence under regulations governing the operation of residential care homes or possibly justification for the cancellation of a Residential Care Home Certificate. However that is a matter for the registration authority of the Residential Care Home and not the DHA.

Premises not registered as nursing homes may be inspected only if there is reasonable cause to suspect that they should be so registered — not that there is reasonable cause to suspect that they are accommodating those who are not receiving adequate care. That is the responsibility of the Social Services Department of the local district or county council as the case may be.

DHAs and their officers should not undertake inspection of non-registered premises without careful consideration and detailed legal advice.

Timing of inspection

In England and Wales inspections can and probably should take place irregularly and at antisocial hours. It is normal practice for one or both of the minimum visits to be arranged by appointment. The purpose of such visits is to check the general operation and fabric and commissioning of the building and to do formal and regular checks on record keeping. There is no point, it is suggested, in arranging such visits without warning as the inspector will need to have close discussions both with the owners and the person in charge. The purpose of the visit will be frustrated if it is not made with a proper appointment. The purpose of an unscheduled visit is quite different. The purpose of that visit is to see what is actually happening at the home at antisocial times when no one has any idea that the visit is expected.

Home owners are reminded that they must give access to a properly authorised inspector and that refusal to give access is a criminal offence and it is the one criminal offence under the legislation governing the registration of nursing homes which may attract a sentence of imprisonment.

There is no justification for the suggestion that in England and Wales inspection must take place at reasonable times.

The DHA inspector must be properly authorised. Curiously he is not required to have any particular qualification or experience. The authority must be in writing and be properly authenticated by the DHA. The written document must state that the inspector is authorised to inspect nursing homes although not, it is suggested, specifically the particular nursing home.

Some home owners have expressed concern in these more violent times that rogues may take advantage of this right of inspection to enter nursing homes at antisocial hours and take advantage of staff or patients. In order to overcome these fears DHAs are recommended to ensure that the document incorporates not only identification of the inspector by name but also a properly authenticated photograph. If trouble is expected or if there is is any particular cause for concern as to the attitude of staff, patients or owners at a particular home, DHAs would do well simply to arrange for an individual letter from the District General Manager to be in the possession of a particular inspector authorising the inspection by reference to place, date and time.

Content of inspection

During the inspection the inspector is entitled to and should look at whatever he or she wishes around and about the nursing home and inspect the records which the nursing home is required to keep or which the nursing home should keep in accordance with good nursing practice. However no one who is not a medical practitioner employed or engaged by the DHA may look at medical records. It is unusual for a medical practitioner to attend routine inspections. There may be grave difficulties in separating medical records from nursing records as in many nursing homes these will be incorporated in the same documentation. However home owners are advised that non-medical practitioners should not be allowed to inspect medical records and DHAs are reminded that their nursing inspectors cannot insist on such inspection.

It is suggested that home owners should not be embarrassed by unenforceable requests and that home owners should not supply the information gratuitously as there may in so doing be a breach of confidence owed to the patient. Confidence is a matter which is the property of the patient concerned and may only be waived by the patient and not by the home owner.

Cancellation of registration

A Certificate of Registration is a permanent certificate. It does not lapse upon expiration of a specified period and it continues unless and until either the home owner ceases to operate a particular nursing home, transfers ownership or it is cancelled by following the appropriate procedures.

There are only two ways to cancel a Certificate of Registration.

- The ordinary method of cancellation as laid out in Sections 31-33 of the 1984 Act.

- The emergency cancellation procedure provided in Section 30 of the 1984 Act.

Grounds for cancellation of registration

As a precondition to cancellation by either method the DHA must be satisfied that grounds for cancellation exist. It will be for the DHA to prove by the civil burden of proof (the balance of probabilities) that such grounds do exist.

Those grounds are set out in Section 28 of the 1984 Act and incorporate by reference the reasons for refusal permitted under Section 25 of the 1984 Act.

The fact that grounds exist does not require the DHA to take action but entitles it to take action if in its discretion it is thought appropriate. If grounds do not exist the DHA has no discretion to take action. A wise

DHA contemplating a proposal to cancel should be sure that if the home owner were to appeal it has a good case to prove the grounds of cancellation before the independent Registered Homes Tribunal. There can be little point in embarking upon cancellation procedure if there is no confidence on the part of the DHA that an appeal could be sustained.

If an application for an emergency cancellation order is to succeed before a magistrate the same grounds must exist but in addition the DHA must show to the magistrate that at the time of the application there will be a serious risk to the life, health or well-being of patients at the home unless the order is made.

Discharge of such a burden of proof is heavy.

An application to the magistrate is not an alternative to the ordinary cancellation procedure and it should only be used where there is genuine evidence of serious risk to patients. It is likely that it will only be in very very unusual and rare cases that such an application is properly made.

It is clearly established on those cases that have come before Registered Homes Tribunals and approved by the decision of the Court of Appeal in Lyons v. East Sussex County Council that if an order is made by a magistrate it may only be sustained on appeal if it is shown that there was evidence and evidence produced to the magistrate of a serious risk to the patients at the date when the application was made.

Magistrate's applications should only be made in a true emergency.

Ordinary procedure for cancellation

Cancellation is a decision for the DHA. The DHA officers will identify grounds which give cause for concern and will no doubt intensify the frequency of inspection and investigation so as to satisfy themselves that their initial suspicions were well founded and that there is a case to be made that for a particular reason (e.g. the fabric of the home, its staffing or the identity of the owners) the conclusion may be formed that the home is no longer fit to operate.

The decision is one for the authority and not the officers.

The procedure is simple and clearly set out in Sections 31-33 of the 1984 Act. Any DHA officer advising upon a prospective cancellation should study those Sections carefully. If the procedure is not followed correctly subsequent proposals and decisions will be held invalid irrespective of merits. There are three steps under the control of the DHA.

- The issue of a written proposal to cancel.
- A consideration of representations (if any) made on behalf of the home owner.
- The formal decision to cancel.

We shall proceed to consider them individually,

Proposal to cancel
Having determined that there are grounds to justify proceedings for

cancellation the DHA by its members and not its officers (although the officers' advice will be crucial) must resolve to make a proposal to cancel the registration. That proposal must be put into writing as a formal Notice specifying the nature of the proposal and the grounds upon which the DHA considers that the cancellation is justified. It will be prudent to refer to the Sections of the 1984 Act under which the proposal is issued and in relation to specific grounds and reasons to refer to the precise statutory reference upon which reliance is made. That Notice must be served upon the home owner and it is very important that the Notice informs the home owner clearly of his right to make representations against the proposal, that right to be notified to the DHA within fourteen days.

Consideration of representations

Before a need to consider representations arises the home owner must have given an indication that he wished to make representations. That indication must be given within fourteen days but it is an indication of an intention to make representations and not the representations themselves. Representations may be in writing or oral and must be made within a reasonable time from the service of the proposal. What is a reasonable time will depend upon the circumstances of a particular case but it is clear that the graver the allegation the shorter the timescale.

A DHA will wish to consider its formal position quickly and it is suggested that it will probably wish to consider the matter at its next full meeting. Therefore it would be prudent when serving a Notice to indicate to the home owner the timing of the DHA's meetings and at that stage to indicate the meeting at which the DHA wishes to consider the matter. Then the home owner will have no opportunity to say that he was not given adequate warning or that the period of time suggested was unreasonable. Whenever considering the reasonableness of any time period one should err on the side of generosity. Remember that if a Court were to find that the period was unreasonable the whole procedure would be nullified.

If the home owner gives notice of intention to make representations and indicates that those representations are in writing the DHA merely awaits their receipt but should specify the timescale within which it expects to receive them. If the home owner indicates that he wishes to make oral representations then the Authority will have to determine the procedure by which it will hear those oral representations. Practices differ. Some DHAs appoint a senior executive officer who has not been concerned with the particular dispute to hear with an independent mind what the home owner has to say. Some DHAs appoint a member of, or an officer from another DHA to hear the representations and make a written report for them at their next meeting. Some DHAs convene a panel consisting of their members either alone or mixed with independent experts. In some cases home owners are invited or requested to call witnesses and present documents and in some cases the owners are instructed that they may only make a simple submission. There are no absolute rules as to the procedure which should be taken.

It is suggested that as it is the home owner who is making the representations he should within reason be permitted to present those oral representations with or without evidence as he sees fit. It is the home owner's case and it is the DHA's duty to hear that case and thus it is suggested that it would be wrong to restrict the manner in which the home owner sought to make his case unless of course the action taken as suggested was unreasonable and time-consuming.

Home owners will face a difficult choice as to whether to make representations and if so whether to make them in writing or orally. Careful consideration will be required and no two cases are the same. It will be a rare case when it would be wise to keep silent, for the right to make representations is a valuable opportunity to head-off time-consuming and costly disputes before the Tribunal. It may be right to limit representations to a written submission where the dispute centres upon different opinions on practice or interpretations of the legislation affecting the operation of the home. Where there are complex disputes as to nursing practice or patient care or where there may be disputes as to the actual facts which have been asserted by the DHA as reported by its officers it may be more appropriate to make oral representations and to tender principals involved for cross-examination by the DHA officers or the investigators so that the DHA in coming to its decision may be fully aware of the other side of the story. One may expect DHAs to support their officers but it is not unusual in a properly conducted enquiry for the initial impression of an officer's report to be shown to be based upon a subjective opinion or to be less grave than appeared from the initial report. Everything will depend upon the circumstances. If there are to be serious disputes on matters of evidence it may well be that the home owner would not wish to reveal the full extent of his case in advance of a Tribunal Hearing as it might be thought that that could give advance warning to witnesses on behalf of the DHA as to the thrust and extent of cross-examination. It is suggested that it would be a rare case in which such considerations are of relevance.

As will be seen in the section on appeals the timescale from the final decision of the Health Authority to the Hearing of a Tribunal will be very short in terms of civil litigation. Therefore those advising home owners themselves should give careful consideration to full preparation for and the delivery of detailed oral representations on the basis that it will either dispose of the case or if the case proceeds to a Tribunal the hard ground work will have been done and the last minute work (always more expensive with the legal profession) or applications for postponements (which are always unwelcome to the Chairmen of Tribunals) may be avoided.

Formal decision to cancel

In making its decision the DHA will carefully consider both the original proposal, subsequent evidence received from the officers and any representations made by the home owner. The DHA should not rubber stamp the original proposal even if no representations are made. It is a clear third step in the procedure to consider the decision. It is suggested that before making a decision there should always have been a further investigation of the facts by the officers. It may well be that the home owner, for reasons of ignorance or perhaps fear of authority, has failed to respond to the Notice formally but has indeed undertaken steps to comply with the DHA complaints. There may be a lively debate before a Tribunal as to the place in time at which the Tribunal is considering facts and matters at the home but it is submitted that debate will be as between the date of the DHA decision and the date of the Tribunal Hearing and will not include the date of the formal proposal. The DHA will have to justify its decision before the Tribunal by reference to the state of fact at the date of its decision. If facts were justified at the date of the proposal but not at the date of the decision then it is unlikely that the DHA will succeed on appeal.

Emergency cancellation

The emergency procedure for cancellation of a Certificate of Registration is set forth in Section 30 of the 1984 Act. This was a new provision in the 1984 Act. It is an extraordinary provision in English Law in that it enables a registering DHA to take away the lawful authority to carry on business from a trader instantaneously without immediate appeal and sometimes without the trader being present. It is a power which must be exercised very carefully.

As has already been shown the DHA will have to demonstrate to the magistrate and will have to justify on appeal that at the date of the Magistrates Court Order there was a serious risk to the health, welfare or safety of patients.

The Order will take effect immediately upon being issued by the magistrate. This is to be contrasted with the ordinary procedure where the Order takes effect only twenty-eight days after the decision or the conclusion of the appeal.

It is submitted that if the correct procedure is not followed precisely then the Magistrates Court Order may be invalid.

The application must be made by a DHA to a magistrate. Again it is the application of the DHA and not the officers. There is no authority but it is suggested that either the DHA or a duly authorised subcommittee of the DHA must formally authorise the application. A decision taken by the officers and an application made without authority would it is suggested be open to challenge.

Evidence must be produced to the magistrate to justify the grounds for cancellation and the gravity of the case. Whether or not the decision is upheld on appeal will depend upon an examination of the reasons given by the magistrate and the magistrate can only give reasons having heard evidence. The Order may be made 'ex parte'. This means that the DHA may apply to the magistrate without warning the home owner. This is a very serious matter. DHAs are recommended to use all efforts in their power to ensure that the home owner knows of the application and is given an opportunity to be present when the application is to be heard. This need not necessarily cause delay. An appointment will have to made with the magistrate and only in rare cases, it is suggested, will it be impossible at least to notify the home owner that the application is being made so that the home owner has an opportunity to be present and to be represented.

DHAs will remember that the Magistrates are not bound to grant the Order. DHAs are not bound to apply ex parte. Magistrates may be more inclined to grant the Order if they know that the home owner has been given the opportunity to appear or if they have heard the home owner and have heard the weakness of his response.

Magistrates are not rubber stamps of the DHA decisions. The magistrate is required to consider the matter and it is the magistrate who must decide from the evidence which he has heard. The application must be supported by a written statement signed by the DHA and it is suggested that it should be signed at the very least by a senior executive officer of the DHA if not the District General Manager. DHAs would seem to be well advised to support that written statement with the presence of witnesses who can tell the magistrate the circumstances and give the magistrate the opportunity to question them. These courses of action whilst not mandatory would it is suggested lead to greater prospects of success in upholding the decision on appeal.

The DHA may wish to ensure that any Order obtained is both valid and likely to be sustained on appeal. Home owners faced with such an Order should carefully consider all the circumstances. The effect of the Order is to cancel the registration. If a DHA or a magistrate were found not to have followed a proper procedure it would be open to the home owner to apply to the High Court for a declaration that the Order was invalid. If the reasons given for the Order fail to show evidence of serious risk to patients or if correct procedures had not been followed it seems likely that the High Court might grant a declaration that the Order was not valid. There is evidence to support the suggestion that even though the application may be made *ex parte* there could be a summons issued and served in the normal way unless a paramount necessity arises. It would seen reasonable that to justify an Order ex parte the DHA would have to show evidence both of serious risk and paramount importance. In the case of Lyons v. East Sussex County Council the Court of Appeal described this Order as draconian. Against that background it is likely that the High Court would favour declaring an Order invalid if they were satisfied that it had been obtained without sufficient evidence, unfairly or without sufficient warning.

An important note should be made for both DHAs and home owners about the effect of a cancellation Order. Cancellation cancels the Certificate and thus cancels the right to carry on the nursing home. The Order does not give legal authority to DHA officers or others to do anything else. No one is entitled to enter premises forcibly. No one is entitled to remove patients forcibly. The image, which has been seen, of a fleet of ambulances engaged by the DHA arriving like the United States

Cavalry at sunrise to rescue the patients of a deregistered home is misconceived.

Such action it is submitted is not justified by law. Once the Order has been made and served upon the home owner the DHA have the same rights and duties as before the service of the Order. They must inspect and must report on further action.

Clearly continuation of the nursing home after a valid Order (and these arguments may only apply to Magistrates Court Orders for Tribunal Orders will have been fully debated) could constitute an offence for which the home owner can and should be prosecuted. Furthermore if the home owner declines to cease operations either of his own volition or in co-operation with the DHA there would be a clear entitlement and indeed a duty on the DHA to seek from the High Court an Injunction to restrain continued operation of the Nursing Home. Failure to comply with that Order, if properly served, would amount to contempt of court and could and would lead to fines, orders for the sequestration of assets and ultimately the committal to prison of those responsible for disobedience.

However DHAs must remember that patients in nursing homes are individuals entitled to the same freedoms as other individuals. Those individuals cannot possibly be removed to other nursing homes, hospitals or places against their wishes. Action can be taken only against the defaulting former home owners.

The DHA would also be able to take the action of reporting nurses, whether owners or employed nurses who continued to operate after a valid Order to their professional body, the United Kingdom Central Council for Nursing and Midwifery. Continuing to nurse patients in premises not registered would surely give rise to a justifiable allegation of professional misconduct on the part of the nurse.

Double procedure

The risks of failing to sustain an Order for Cancellation made under Section 30 of the 1984 Act by a failure of evidence of serious risk were canvassed and recognised by the Court of Appeal in Lyons v. East Sussex County Council. The Court saw that there might very well be a case where an appeal would be upheld because of insufficient evidence of serious risk at the date when the Order was made but the Tribunal might feel that a Cancellation Order would have been justified under the ordinary proce-dure in any event. If only a Magistrates Court Order existed and there were no ordinary cancellation procedure before the Tribunal, the Tribunal would then be obliged to to allow the appeal. That would clearly be an unsatisfactory position and the Court of Appeal has given express approval to the practice whereby an ordinary cancellation procedure could be followed simultaneously with an appeal against a Magistrates Court Order.

There may still be technical difficulties and DHAs should take careful legal advice as to the timing of their procedures. It is suggested that it is unlikely that an emergency would arise with such suddenness that there had not been previous concern and it is recommended that the ordinary procedure be started before an application for an emergency Order. If the ordinary procedure is begun after the Magistrates Court Order then it is open to the criticism that it is nullity. If the Magistrates Court Order is valid there would be no Certificate to cancel if the Decision is made after the Order it would have to rely on different evidence. DHAs should take their legal advice very carefully when making any decisions about an Emergency Closure Order under Section 30 of the 1984 Act.

Appeals

The appeal system from DHA decisions was revolutionised by the 1984 Act.

Before, appeals were heard in the Magistrates Court. This was unsatisfactory because in many cases matters of nursing practice and technical issues relating to the structure and operation of nursing homes fell to be determined by stipendiary or lay magistrates who probably had no prior relevant experience. Further, rightly or wrongly, appellants felt themselves disadvantaged as they foresaw that the magistrates would tend to accept the professional and technical evidence given on behalf of the health authority thus adopting the very position of health authority officers whose judgment might have been at the very centre of the items in dispute.

The Registered Homes Tribunal is truly independent. Each Tribunal is convened especially for the particular case. There is a panel of part-time Chairmen and professional non-legal members who are selected to deal with each case. In addition to the legally qualified Chairmen there will be a doctor and a nurse. The Tribunal will have no connection whatsoever with the health authority and listen carefully to both sides of the argument.

Home owners will always be the Appellants because there will only be an appeal against a decision adverse to the home owner. Home owners need have no fear that their case will not be heard impartially by the Tribunal.

In delivering its formal decision a health authority must give notice of the right of appeal and Notice of Appeal is given to the health authority. The writer suggests that a copy of that Notice always be sent to the Registered Homes Tribunal Secretariat to avoid delays and confusions if, as has occurred, the authority officials delay or forget to transmit the appeal. Notice of Appeal is simple. It merely requires statement of an intention to appeal. It must be delivered within twenty-eight days after receipt of the Decision. There is no power to extend the time other then by agreement and one cannot imagine that a health authority would willingly agree to an extension. If the time is missed the appeal will be lost.

The Registered Homes Tribunal is a legal Tribunal and will hear evidence both as to the facts and from experts. It will consider submissions on law and make rulings based upon its findings on the law and will reach a decision upon the view that it has taken of the facts.

All those concerned with the Tribunal must appreciate its legal nature. It is not necessary to be represented by a lawyer but it is recommended that such representation is sought. The Tribunals are conducted formally and evidence will have to be presented and cross-examined in a formal way. The strict rules of Court will not apply but the Chairman will be assiduous to ensure in a spirit of fair play that each side is aware of the other's case and that normal rules of evidence are followed unless there are very good reasons for him to exercise his discretion to permit the variation therefrom.

Registered Homes Tribunals are likely to take many days and in some cases many weeks, if there are many and complex issues of fact. Health authority managers and their advisers considering an Appeal should seriously take into account both the legal cost of preparation and representation and the hidden cost of lost man hours in executives and witnesses attending the Hearing. Once an Appeal has been lodged the Tribunal will expect the matter to be dealt with quickly. It is said that the Tribunals expect a Hearing to begin nine weeks from the date of service of the Notice of Appeal with a decision given a few weeks after the conclusion of the Hearing. This time-table cannot be met on some occasions where cases are lengthy or complex but experience shows that Tribunal Chairmen are wholly unsympathetic to repeated requests for adjournments and that lack of sympathy applies equally both to Appellants and Respondents. The Tribunal seems to take the view that the parties should know and have prepared their case prior to the health authority decision and there should be no reason for lengthy delays for evidence gathering or preparation.

A tight schedule is provided for formal preparation of a Tribunal case.

Not less than thirty days before the Hearing the health authority must prepare and serve on the Tribunal and the Appellant a detailed statement of the reasons for its decision.

This should be a simple statement from which the Tribunal and the Appellant can understand the points which the authority proposes to prove and the Appellant will have to meet. It is a matter of regret that even in extended cases authorities appear to see a tactical advantage in waiting until the very last minute to serve these reasons. Appellant's advisers should not be slow to criticise and to chase, for, until the statement of reasons is delivered, the Appellant's solicitor cannot begin properly to prepare all of his case.

Nine days later, no later than twenty-one days before the Hearing the Appellant must file the grounds of appeal. These rules are set out in the RHT Rules.

Tribunal Chairmen have developed further rules of practice. It is obviously inconvenient for either side to be taken by surprise by documents, allegations or evidence brought in at the last minute. Therefore the Tribunal Chairmen have decided that there should be an exchange of evidence in affidavit or statement form and documents upon which reliance is to be placed, no later than fourteen days before the Hearing and that wherever possible an agreed bundle of such documents should be supplied to the Tribunal.

Proper attention to the preparation of the Statement of Reasons, the grounds of appeal and the evidence and the documents may shorten the Tribunal Hearing itself for the Tribunal as well as the parties will be thoroughly conversant with the issues.

Both sides must remember that under no circumstances can either be ordered to pay the costs of the other. Therefore if either party behaves capriciously, either withdraws at the last minute or has its case wholly rejected there is no remedy in costs. This must be borne in mind most carefully by all advising in relation to prospective appeals.

Health authorities have to bear in mind possible waste of their valuable financial resources and home owners find the costs of an appeal, even if successful, a considerable burden. There are a number of very good licence protection legal fee insurance schemes available and home owners should carefully investigate such matters with their insurance brokers. The premiums are low and though cover may be rather limited, will give protection against the really heavy costs of a contested Tribunal Hearing which may arise for any home owner at any time.

At the hearing before the Registered Homes Tribunal the burden of proof will lie upon the health authority in most cases. That means that the health authority must satisfy the Tribunal upon the balance of probabilities that the decision which it has made was made upon proper legal grounds and was justified. If the health authority fails to discharge the burden of proof then the appeal will succeed.

Before embarking on the costly process of an appeal, advisers to health authorities are recommended seriously to consider all the issues in the case and seriously to evaluate whether they will succeed before the Tribunal. There may be difficulties as certain officers may feel that homes should be run in accordance with their dictates or opinions. It is not the opinion of the officers or the health authority which will concern the Tribunal, it is for the Tribunal to decide if the health authority has made a correct decision based on legal grounds. Grounds for refusal or cancellation of Registration are limited by the 1984 Act and the grounds as specified in the Act will be restrictively interpreted. The health authority must show not that their officer's opinion is bona fide or well founded but that the cause of complaint is such as to justify refusal or cancellation of the Registration.

The writer feels that a proper legal analysis of the issues at an early stage will lead to many potential Appeals being abandoned. The Registered Homes Tribunal is sole judge of fact. The Appeal process will be over when the decision is published and if the decision is adverse to the home the matter will be closed and if that involves cancellation of Registration that cancellation will take effect from publication of the decision. There is thus a 'sudden death' conclusion and home owners engaged in such cancellation procedures must appreciate in advance the risks and should make contingency plans for losing. Continuation of the home after a cancellation decision is unlawful and the owner might be prosecuted for a criminal offence. It is prudent for discussions to taken place before the decision as to what steps will be taken in relation to patients should the decision prove adverse. If the home owner succeeds the contingency plans may be shelved but distress and disaster may follow if the matter has not been addressed.

After the decision of the Registered Homes Tribunal there may be a further Appeal to the High Court but not on questions of fact. The High Court will only hear questions of law and an Appeal to the High Court does not have the effect, save by agreement, of suspending or delaying the effect of the Order for Cancellation of the Registration. If the home owner wishes to assert that the Tribunal got the facts wrong they will have to go so far as to say that no reasonable Tribunal could have come to the conclusion reached. That will be an almost impossible burden and it is suggested that the High Court will almost never intervene in what is an expert judgment made by experts appointed to hear this type of factual dispute.

There is no procedure for determining issues of law in advance of the Hearing of the Registered Tribunal but Tribunal Chairmen are not unsympathetic to an early application for a preliminary hearing if there is a serious issue. The writer suggests that home owner advisers should quickly identify any important issues of law which may affect the final result and seek to have those rulings made prior to the full hearing of the Tribunal so that if the ruling is adverse the party concerned may apply to the High Court for a further Appeal and seek to adjourn the main Tribunal Hearing. This avoids the difficulty of a Tribunal deciding to cancel registration with disastrous consequences to the home where a later ruling of the High Court is that that ruling is flawed in law. A particular problem will face a health authority and a Tribunal in a case where an Emergency Closure Order has been obtained from a magistrate. In order to succeed on appeal in upholding the Closure Order from a magistrate the authority must show that there was a serious risk to patients at the time when the Order was made. Thus it may be that the Tribunal is constrained to allow the appeal although it feels that the registration would have been cancelled under the ordinary procedure because of deficiencies in the home which did not amount to a proven serious risk to patients. Such a situation was presented to the Court of Appeal in Lyons v. East Sussex County Council and the Court of Appeal expressly approved the policy of Registration Authorities proceeding with the two separate procedures simultaneously. The Tribunal may hear two appeals together and it is clearly sensible to have both the appeal against the Closure Order of the Magistrate and an appeal against cancellation by the ordinary process heard together.

A further difficulty will be presented in the case of a home which is the subject of a cancellation decision from a health authority where steps have been taken to correct all the defects which justify cancellation prior to the Hearing of the Tribunal but after the published decision of the health authority. The question arises as to whether the Tribunal is to consider the matter as at the date when the health authority made its decision or as at the date of the Tribunal Hearing. Opinions differ and there is no authority on the point from the High Court. In a recent case a Tribunal upheld the submission from the authority that the Tribunal being an Appeal Tribunal could only consider facts at the date of the health authority decision. The Tribunal expressly approved the procedure adopted by the Appellant, in that case at the suggestion of the Respondent, where the Appellant had during the course of the Appeal lodged a new application for registration for determination by the health authority and the Tribunal adjourned the hearing until determination by the health authority of the new application so that the two appeals could be heard together (if necessary) and then the Tribunal would be able to consider the situation at the home at the date of the second decision. Indeed both appeals might be found unnecessary if the authority agreed with the Appellant that matters had been put right.

That procedure seems sensible and merely involves the Appellant in payment of a new Registration fee (considerably less than the costs of an appeal to the High Court where there is a risk of paying the costs of the other side if one loses) and avoids lengthy, bruising, costly and possibly unnecessary hearings before a Tribunal.

Home owners are recommended in cases where alleged defects have been corrected, following a health authority decision, to lodge an immediate new application accompanied by the appropriate fee and seek an adjournment of the outstanding appeal pending determination of that application.

8 Health care trends

Ben Thomas

Health care as an industry is rapidly developing and changing. Advances in medical technology result in both more 'high technology' and, equally, more less-invasive procedures.

Managers need to be alert to trends in care and to new developments. This chapter covers screening, occupational health and rehabilitation, which are all growing activities, with much further potential.

Traditionally hospitals have provided a facility to enable consultants to see patients referred to them by other doctors. The trend is now to look for other sources of business, including direct sales by the hospital to patients and other services which involve selling products to corporate customers.

Introduction

Throughout the 1980s hospitals and nursing homes have witnessed a gradual but continuing reduction in the length of inpatient stay. This reduction has been brought about by a combination of factors.

First, some of the advances in medical techniques and technology. A good example is lithotripsy — a technique used to break up and remove kidney stones non-invasively. Conventional surgery involves a two-week stay in hospital followed by up to a six-week period of convalescence. However, with lithotripsy the overall treatment time is reduced to three or four days and in some cases the procedure can now be undertaken on an outpatient basis.

The second reason is the pressure exerted by the third-party insurers who in order to minimise the cost of policies based on claims-related experience have encouraged people to be treated on a shorter stay or day basis wherever this is practicable.

The third reason is patient pressure. Patients want to be treated quickly and return to normal activity as soon as possible.

The reduction in patient stay has focused the attention of the owners and managers of independent hospitals and nursing homes on new services, alternative sources of revenue and encouraged them to look at health-care provision in its broader sense. The importance of revenue generation from day care, pathology, physiotherapy and radiology is already well accepted and in many cases now forms a major part of total revenue.

There are, however, other services which are now featuring more prominently in planning for the future and these include health screening, occupational health and rehabilitation. In this chapter these services are examined in relation to the place they occupy in the independent sector, their likely development and the possible effect the NHS review may have.

Health screening

Health screening in its purest sense is a technique employed by physicians in looking for detectable diseases or physiological change amongst the population. The term, however, has become more popularly associated in the UK with executive health screening or health assessment which has traditionally been aimed at those people in social categories A and B aged 35 to 64.

Executive screening was introduced into the UK at a corporate level by the Institute of Directors in the 1960s. This particular unit was taken over by BUPA in 1971 and from this modest start BUPA Medical Centres developed to become the largest corporate provider of screening services in Western Europe. Today this company has twenty-four static centres and ten mobile units. The latest published figures show that the company screened over 100,000 men and women during 1988.

Five years ago a small number of corporate providers including PPP, BUPA and AMI enjoyed a virtual monopoly of the screening market. Today, the situation is very different with over one hundred and fifty organisations throughout the UK involved in screening with nearly a third of these based in London and the South East. A recent review of screening units in Central London showed that just over 30 per cent of the units are based in independent hospitals.

Screening is certainly not new. Antenatal care has been around a long time and mass radiography was used extensively to detect tuberculosis until the incidence of the disease was not sufficient to warrant the high cost of screening. In the 1980s the two leading killers have been cancers and heart disease. These are the main targets of screening services. An increased knowledge of the risk factors together with improved screening techniques means that the medical world is far better equipped to combat these diseases.

But why has there been such a dramatic increase in the number of screening units? The reasons are many and complex but can be summarised as:

• Health care has become a much more important issue on the political agenda, media coverage has been extensive and companies and individuals are far more aware and concerned about health and related issues.

- Organisations and companies have become increasingly convinced of the importance of providing health care services such as health insurance and health screening to their senior staff.

- Independent hospitals have realised that they can provide screening facilities at very little extra cost, therefore, they can operate on a marginal basis and achieve good commercial returns. Screening patients in hospital also generates extra inpatient and outpatient activity as a result of problems diagnosed during the screening process.

This last reason is important and holds the key to why so many screening facilities are located in independent hospitals. Traditionally health screening for men and women has involved a doctor taking a detailed medical history and undertaking a full physical examination. This has been accompanied by a range of tests; chest X-ray, lung function, hearing and vision, urinalysis, biochemistry, cervical smear and mammography and here of course hospitals have a number of advantages over dedicated screening centres.

- The high cost of specialist equipment required for screening, for example X-ray equipment can be shared between various departments in the hospital.

- Diagnostic tests can be undertaken by the pathology and radiology departments at very little extra cost using existing equipment.

- Staffing can be minimised and shared, for example receptionists and nursing.

The NHS has always viewed screening as an obvious method of generating income and recent enquiries revealed that over twenty five health authorities are attempting to sell screening services to companies and organisations in their catchment areas.

The Forrest Report published in 1987 acted as the catalyst for authorities to organise breast screening centres. Other initiatives have been put forward by the Government to improve facilities for screening of cervical cancer.

The major problem in both areas would appear to be funding rather than commitment on the part of the NHS. More recently general practitioners have also been encouraged to undertake some screening although at a more basic level, for example blood pressure and cholesterol checks.

Health screening will continue to develop in the independent sector. Convenient appointment times, quick reliable reporting systems and pleasant surroundings are important and valued by customers. The range and flexibility of services offered will grow and will encompass such areas as endoscopy screening for the early detection of bowel disease, psychometric testing and individual packages tailored to meet the needs of organisations.

The activities of screening centres do, however, need to be monitored to ensure that the high standards established are maintained over the coming years. In June 1989 the independent sector launched a code of practice covering 200 independent screening centres throughout the UK. This is a first step but there is still a need for a statutory licensing authority, independent of the operators, which would inspect and accredit centres.

Occupational health

Unlike health screening the market for occupational health services relates far more closely to the work-force and the delivery of services may well take place almost exclusively at the place of work rather than in an off-site medical facility. Before describing how services are provided in the UK it is important to understand the functions of an occupational health service. The most effective way to do this is by quoting directly from an International Labour Organisation convention (ILO, 1985) which summarised the functions of an occupational health service as:

* Identification and assessment of the risks from health hazards in the work-place.

* Surveillance of the factors in the working environment and working practices which may affect worker's health, including sanitary installations, canteens and housing where these facilities are provided by an employer.

* Advice on planning and organisation of work, including the design of work-places, on the choice, maintenance and condition of machinery and other equipment and on substances used in work.

* Participation in the development of programmes for the testing of working practices as well as testing and evaluation of health aspects of new equipment.

* Advice on occupational health, safety and hygiene and ergonomics and individual and collective protective equipment.

* Surveillance of worker's health in relation to work.

* Promoting the adaptation of work to the worker.

* Contribution of means of vocational rehabilitation

* Collaboration in providing information, training and education in the fields of occupational health, hygiene and ergonomics.

* Organising of first aid and emergency treatment.

* Participation in analysis of occupational accidents and occupational diseases.

It is interesting to note that after several years of consultation the Health and Safety Executive announced in December 1988 'We advise the Government that no decision should be taken on ratification at this stage but the position should be reviewed in three years'.

During the past twenty-five years occupational health services in the UK have almost exclusively been provided by companies in the independent sector. The NHS has introduced local services for its own staff but until recently had rarely offered services to outside organisations. The market is currently dominated by four groups: general practitioners of whom there are thought to be some 2000 working part-time; in-house occupational health services such as British Telecom and Shell, Group Services; charitable or guarantee companies set up in the 1960s and 1970s with money from the Nuffield Foundation; and the health care providers including AMI, BUPA and PPP who have entered the market in the last three years.

As can be seen from Table 8.1 the corporate providers do not include any independent hospital operators, other than AMI and BUPA but it should be noted that even in the case of these two groups the hospitals are only used as bases for the occupational health teams and for undertaking some health screening when access to diagnostic facilities is required.

The vast majority of occupational health services can be and are provided in the work-place. These include pre-employment health screening, health surveillance programmes, health and safety audits, ergonomic surveys and health promotion.

An analysis of the financial results of the companies in Table 8.1 reveals that although the majority are making a modest surplus some are still sustaining losses. Indeed a group service which has been operating for over twenty years reported a loss of £80,000 on a turnover of £500,000 in the year to August 1988. The health care organisations such as AMI, BUPA and PPP consolidate their accounts within the group accounts so it is difficult to assess their progress to date.

There are increasing pressures on organisations to provide professional occupational health care for their staff. This pressure comes from legislation and new codes of practice, for example the new control of substances hazardous to health regulations which come into force in October 1989 and new hearing regulations which come into force in 1990. There is also a growing awareness and recognition by organisations that the management of employee health in the workplace is primarily a management task and one which can have a significant effect on the performance of business.

Today occupational health care is mainly found in larger or potentially dangerous organisations which employ at the most seven million of the UK's total work force. The remaining twenty million have no more than the facilities required by the Health and Safety at Work Act (First Aid Regulations) 1981.

So how will the occupational-health companies respond to the steady but increasing need to provide services, how will they be marketed, what if any are the opportunities for the independent hospitals and how will the NHS perform?

Occupational-health companies will continue to provide a range of core services and to market and sell these in order to :

Table 8.1 Occupational health companies

Company/Organisation	Geographical area covered
AMI	UK
AMARC	North East
Aycliffe OHS	County Durham
BUPA	UK
Central Middlesex OHS	West London
GKN	Midlands
Harlow OHS	Harlow and surrounding district
Institute of OH (Birmingham)	UK
Kings Lynn OHS	East Anglia
Lifewatch (Scotland)	Glasgow and Edinburgh
Midlands OHS	Birmingham
Milton Keynes	Milton Keynes
Mobile Audiometric Services	UK
Northern Industrial Health Services	Newcastle
Offshore Medical Services	Aberdeen and offshore oil fields
PPP	UK
Rochdale	Rochdale
School of Tropical Hygiene and Medicine	UK
Southern Counties (Guildford)	Surrey
Slough OHS	Slough and surrounding district
Telford and District OHS	Telford

- Promote, protect, restore and maintain the good health and well-being of all employees in the work-place.
- Promote and enhance the image of organisations as caring and responsible employers thereby enabling them to attract and retain the right staff.
- Reduce the financial impact of illness throughout organisations thereby increasing productivity and profitability.

In order to meet these criteria occupational-health providers will need experienced and qualified staff who can audit the health-care needs of organisations and provide cost-effective solutions to comply with both the statutory and budgetary requirements of companies. This requirement for specialist staff will mean that the dedicated companies will continue to provide core occupational-health services with the independent hospitals and screening centres concentrating on the more financially attractive health screening market. Some of the occupational-health companies already provide executive screening and view this as an activity which allows them to produce a surplus or profit.

The NHS has seized upon occupational-health care as a major opportunity but like a number of other organisations health authorities regard screening and occupational health as synonymous. The NHS must, however, be seen as a threat in view of its low cost base and its ability to use its localised marketing within business communities to sell its services commercially whilst enabling the local companies to support the NHS. A number of authorities are already promoting themselves and the West Lambeth Health Authority has recently won two major contracts, one with the Greater London Fire and Civil Defence Authority, the second with the Foreign and Commonwealth Office.

Rehabilitation

In 1972 the Mair Report defined rehabilitation as the 'restoration of patients to their full physical, mental and social capability' (Scottish Home and Health Department), and this remains one of the widest accepted definitions. In 1980 the World Health Organisation published the international classification of impairments, disability and handicaps which distinguishes between 'impairment disability and handicap as different dimensions of the consequence of disease'.

A more recent definition is 'the management of disability' that is the identification and management of problems caused by disability, by the utilisation of services which aim to minimise care and dependency and to maximise social opportunity and independence.

Two reports published in 1972, the Mair Report in Scotland and the Tunbridge Report in England (DHSS) pointed the way ahead for rehabilitation services. Rehabilitation centres vary greatly in size and method of operation. Some centres were developed during the first and second World Wars, such as Oswestry Orthopaedic Hospital and the Bridge of Earn Hospital in Perthshire, Scotland. Centres continued to develop in a piecemeal fashion until in 1975 the Minister of Health designated twelve centres as demonstration centres. These have now grown to twenty-nine covering a wide range of specialities from child and adult rehabilitation, neurological disorders, geriatric rehabilitation and cardiac rehabilitation. All of these centres operate within the NHS.

In the independent sector there have been a few developments, notably Unstead Park in Surrey, a general rehabilitation centre run by the Nestor Group, and two units for head injuries in Northamptonshire, the Kemsley Unit at St Andrews Hospital and Grafton Manor run by AMI. The newest unit which opened in 1988, is the Devonshire Hospital in central London which was converted from an acute facility and is run by the St Martins Group.

The main source of statistical data concerning the incidence of disability in the UK is the Harris report published in 1971. This showed that there were just over three million people, aged 16 and over, with some form of physical or mental or sensory impairment. Ten per cent of disabled people are aged over 45, 30 per cent are between 46 and 64 and 60 per cent are 65 or over. Disability is therefore prevalent in the elderly population and is mainly associated with geriatric services.

The principal causes of severe physical disability are neurological disorders. In the average health district with a population of 250,000 there will be a minimum of 200 disabled patients with multiple sclerosis, 500 people with Parkinsonism of whom 55 will be severely disabled. There will be 1800 wheelchair users and about 11,000 people will suffer urinary incontinence.

There may also be up to 6,000 people diagnosed as having rheumatoid arthritis although some of these will not necessarily be disabled.

In the UK private health care is currently funded by health insurance or by individuals paying directly for treatment. In order to cover rehabilitation services new insurance policies may have to be produced. There are also a significant number of personal injury and permanent health insurance claims requiring rehabilitation services and it would be feasible for the insurance companies to pay this direct.

Some health authorities already contract out some of the rehabilitation services to the independent sector. This is particularly attractive where health authorities have only very few patients and setting up a separate service would be very expensive. Voluntary societies and charities might also consider giving financial backing to services which they can see to be beneficial to their members.

A number of independent hospitals already provide cardiac rehabilitation services which because they are expensive to set up are usually organised as part of a full cardiac programme. Sports injuries are far more common and are often run as an extension of the physiotherapy department.

Other areas which could be considered in the future include a rehabilitation advisory service, counselling services for the management of breast disease, incontinence advisory service and domiciliary rehabilitation.

The future

Predicting the future of health care in the United Kingdom is not an easy exercise, much will depend upon a continuing stable political situation and how quickly the recommendations contained in the recently published White Paper are implemented. What is apparent is that organisations rather than individual hospitals and nursing homes will play an increasingly important role in the delivery of health-care services within the independent sector.

The independent sector has been in the forefront of health screening and occupational health over the past twenty years. That position is now beginning to be challenged by the NHS with the advent of general management, hospitals opting out and a genuine commercial awareness. The challenge may simply mean existing business being transferred between providers in the two sectors or a massive increase in the market.

Whatever happens the future for health care is not going to be dull!

References

DHSS Central Health Services Council 1972 *Rehabilitation*. HMSO (Tunbridge Report)

Harris AI 1971 *Handicapped and impaired in Great Britain*. HMSO (Harris Report)

ILO 1985 *Convention 161*. International Labour Organisation

Scottish Home and Health Department. Scottish Health Service Council 1972 *Medical Rehabilitation*. HMSO Edinburgh ('Mair Report')

WHO 1980 *International classification of impairments, disabilities and handicaps*. World Health Organisation Geneva

9 Partnership and competition with the NHS

Haydn Cook

The NHS is still our 'big brother', and no book of this sort would be complete without a mention of the overlap. With the Review of the NHS, it is evident that the whole form of health care may change over the next few years. The writer reviews the present situation, and makes some informed guesses regarding the future.

History

When the NHS was created in the early post-war period, a few hospitals were exempted from the legislation. Until the 'Barbara Castle' Labour Government of the 1970s the private sector was a small residual sector of mainly charitable and religious-based units.

Barbara Castle, in an attempt to drive 'pay beds' out of the NHS, inadvertently created a thriving and rapidly growing private sector. From being a poor relation, it became a still small, but thrusting industry. It was, at the same time, supported by the rapid growth in private medical insurance, and a growth in the number of insurers.

By the early 1980s the private or independent sector had become well established. 'Going private' was an established and now accepted practice, and the private sector had become so large that it was unlikely that any government could destroy it. Whilst the private sector grew in confidence, there was still a considerable gulf between it and the NHS.

Income generation

Two major events during the 1980s have led to greater overlap and integration between the two sectors. First the introduction of Griffiths-style general management has consciously sought to bring to the NHS a more commercial approach and attitude.

Secondly, the Government established the process of 'contracting out' of services. They had felt that 'in-house' hotel services should be exposed to competition, and achieved this by requiring authorities to consider bids for cleaning and other services from outside companies.

This had two implications. First that the service had to be closely specified to prepare the tender document, which resulted inevitably in a detailed review of the service. Secondly, the 'in-house' bid was often based on a streamlined service, so, although they might win the contract and remain an 'in-house' service, it was often on the basis of reduced costs.

Following on from the 'contracting out' exercise, the Conservative Government has demanded that the NHS units should endeavour to generate significant income from local commercial opportunities. Whilst this may not have had much real impact in revenue terms, it has greatly changed the culture within the NHS, with many General Managers now being more sensitive to commercial considerations, and looking for revenue-generating opportunities. Not only have they wanted to learn from the experience of the private sector, but they have also looked at the private sector as a possible source of revenue. Such schemes have included a mish-mash of ideas, including developing shopping malls, offering advertising facilities and selling training services.

Cynics might observe that the only 'commercialisation' of the NHS is the enthusiasm for higher salaries, business cards and employer-provided cars (even if with the latter you have to pay for them!), but the reality is that there has been a fundamental shift in attitude. From viewing the private sector with some disdain, General Managers now have considerable respect for their opposite numbers, and a greater willingness to act as equals. I will cover later in this chapter the ways in which income generation schemes have led to co-operation and joint ventures between the two sectors.

The NHS has been keen to develop the use of pay beds to generate more revenue. Until the recent Medicines Act, in theory they should only be allowed to cover their costs, but at the very least it was hoped, and felt, that they could make a contribution towards covering general overheads. These clearly compete with the private-sector beds, and have some significant competitive advantages. In particular, they have better access to general NHS clinical back-up facilities, sophisticated diagnostic services, and so on. They are also very convenient for the consultant.

However, to date, few Districts have achieved an acceptable standard of hotel services to support these private patients, and have failed to appreciate the real needs of these patients. Also, the government has been reluctant to fund improvements to pay beds, when other priorities exist. There is also an inherent problem, in that the obvious course of action is to use existing diagnostic and other facilities for private patients. As a result, these private patients are perceived as 'queue jumping'. However, the shared costs do mean that the pay beds will always be able to undercut the private sector, but are unlikely to offer an equal service.

Private sector managers have been worried that good NHS General Managers could potentially compete very effectively, and the review may encourage this trend. However, equally it is doubtful whether, for the next two years, they will have any time to devote to pay beds, with all the other urgent priorities. No doubt the pay beds will therefore live on, as a second-rate kind of private-patient bed used by doctors with Medical School rather than NHS contracts which prevent them working 'off site', where there are particular advanced facilities, and by those patients who are particularly cost conscious.

To date, pay beds have been perceived as very profitable (in the sense of contributing towards overheads), but once there are proper costing procedures, including capital costs, and private patients in the NHS are fully costed, I believe that there will be a greater appreciation that, as in private hospitals, it is difficult to make even a 10 per cent profit margin. At that stage, NHS managers will realise that pay beds are in a way a peripheral consideration, and certainly not one which will have a vast impact on the financial viability of the NHS.

NHS review

The Review arose from a period of concern regarding the NHS, partly about a lack of resources and long waiting lists, and in part due to a general concern that the NHS was no longer providing the kind of service required by the general public. The report, published in early 1989, concentrates on making the NHS more consumer-orientated, and proposes the separation of funding (although still through taxation), and provision of health care. Crucially however, care will remain free at the point of delivery.

Some hospitals will be encouraged to become self-governing trusts in an attempt to bring improvements through more local management, and these hospitals will be competing for NHS patients and funds. The definition of 'self-governing' has caused some confusion and concern. Whilst it is intended that they should be 'independent', they will remain within the NHS.

The Review does not propose an increase in funds, but I believe that people's expectations of better services, and competition between units based on quality of service, will cause a substantial increase in the cost of the NHS.

The review will result in the NHS hospitals becoming more like private units, in a number of ways. First, they will have to provide better financial information regarding costs, and will have to price their various services. Capital assets, from land and equipment down to items, or sets of items, of a value of over £1,000 will be charged to the accounts, in the way in which rent and depreciation have always hit private hospital accounts. Rough estimates indicate that selling prices will have to rise by over 10 per cent to cover the cost of capital.

Competition for contracts from funding authorities will result in a marketing and sales function similar to that in the private sector. Large GP practices will also have budgets to buy services, and will therefore be a marketing target.

There is some expectation that the self-governing trust hospitals will be competing with the private hospitals for business. At the same time the private hospitals may obtain NHS contracts. Whilst in principle this may happen, the real issue is whether they will both offer the same level of service.

Many industries offer two or more standards of service, such as 'Business Class' flights and hotels, particularly, offer a varying number of 'stars', with variable prices. I believe that it is likely there will continue to be a 'general' standard of care and a 'higher' grade. It may well be that both offer similar clinical care, but that the latter will offer, for example, a definite admission date, and a single room. It is likely that government funds will cover the more basic service and that insurance and 'self pay' will cover the latter. Within self-governing units it may be easier to buy an 'upgrade' but it is likely that there will continue to be the distinctive styles of service offered in separate units by government and private hospitals. However, there is little doubt that the gulf between the two sectors will be narrowed, with a more nearly continuous spectrum of services available.

Ironically, the commercialisation of the NHS over recent years has been perceived to be a considerable threat to the private sector. General Managers have been keen to upgrade pay beds, to generate revenue, and they are potentially a serious threat to the private sector.

The Review, with its short and intensive time-table of change, means that General Managers will almost certainly be distracted from the pay beds issue, as they are under great pressure to reorganise again, and sort out the 'public' beds as opposed to the, relatively few, pay beds.

Waiting list initiatives

Over the last few years the Government has tried to reduce the NHS waiting lists by the injection of earmarked cash. Regions and Districts have been encouraged to reduce the length of specific lists, in co-operation with the surgeons concerned.

One option has been to ask local private hospitals to bid for the work, another has been to do the work 'in-house'. The attraction of the former is a definite commitment to do the work. The latter is theoretically the cheaper, since, given spare capacity, the NHS can do the work simply at the marginal cost of the staff concerned.

Using private units has run into a number of difficulties. In particular it has been necessary to deal with the question of clinical responsibility and professional fees. Many doctors are unwilling for others to be involved in clearing their lists — equally some have not been willing to do extra work to clear their own lists without extra payment, and authorities have been reluctant to meet this request. Other problems have involved patients who have been unwilling to meet the extra cost of transport to a local, but less immediate, private unit, and similar minor but complicating problems. There have been a number of more general difficulties, in particular, the unpredictability of the amount of money available, or its timing. This has resulted in many wasted bids, followed by a mad rush to spend money, where the main criterion has suddenly become the ability to carry out volumes of work at short notice.

All in all it has not been a great success in terms of numbers of patients dealt with, but it has certainly reduced waiting lists by determining whether those that are apparently 'waiting' are really still on the list! In the context of the Review, it would be inadvisable to be unduly optimistic regarding the possibility of obtaining work from the NHS if this experience is any indicator.

Cross selling of services

In theory, it should be possible for the NHS to sell substantial volumes of services to the private sector, and for the private sector to sell back its own expertise.

The NHS has the advantage of size, and great economies of scale in terms of technological procedures, purchasing, and in many other ways. General Managers have been keen to sell services, often with the view that any price above the marginal cost is making a contribution to overheads; some have almost appeared to believe that any revenue is to the good, and that the costs can always be lost somewhere!

Obvious services to sell have included laundry and pathology. There is no doubt that the NHS could achieve the required standard of service, and the price. However, the private sector have been worried about the industrial relations implication, which to a degree, is a hangover from the 1970s. Their fear has been that, given any industrial strife, the private work would be 'blacked', a risk not worth taking — continuity of standards and service being crucial. Other services have included fire and security advice, and physiotherapy and pharmacy support.

Only limited progress has been made in such sales: I suspect that NHS managers will need to get a convincing commitment from their own staff regarding industrial action before such sales will develop. With regard to some services, it may be that quality is also an issue, where, for example, it is thought that hotel-type commercial laundries will better match the private requirement.

Private units have less scope to sell services, and usually, are organised on a small scale to meet their own demand only. Typically the management structure is relatively tight, and concentrating on their own management problems is sufficient, without taking on the extra demands of obtaining and running contracts. One particular opportunity is the sale of cook-chill or cook-freeze food to health authorities, subject to the achievement of particularly high standards in view of problems and scares. Such suppliers may of course come from catering and hotel operations rather than private health care.

Long-stay sector

Much of the interest in the private sector concentrates on the acute sector, and the long-stay sector is much neglected. It exists in two major elements, the larger of which is the accommodation provided by private nursing homes and the other has many beds, often charitably run, for the chronically ill, the handicapped and the terminally ill.

Private nursing homes now provide roughly half the beds for the elderly. Residential homes, which provide related care, now have more beds in the private sector than are provided by local authorities. Many of these beds offer a contract service to the NHS either on a per patient basis, or on a per bed basis. This area of activity is likely to continue to grow, at least in line with the size of the ageing population. Domiciliary care, including nursing and physiotherapy, is also likely to continue to expand.

Joint ventures

Most recently, joint ventures have become popular, where the common denominator is the private sector's ability to raise capital more easily and on a commercial basis. Two approaches have been evident, the first being where the NHS offers land, in some form, to a developer, as a pay-off for capital development. This arrangement can, in principle, enable the District Health Authority (DHA) to obtain the building it needs quickly, in return for land made available in the future. Usually such land will be for housing or other development purpose, and some discount will be included to cover the private company's cost of interim finance.

Bromley Health Authority, for example, have been keen to trade the development of a new hospital for land with residential development potential. In principle this is a straightforward proposition, but it is facing some objections, especially from the Treasury. International Hospitals Group and McAlpine are the proposed private sector partners.

The other scheme is one where private units, such as day units or private beds are built on hospital land. The theory is that the NHS gets access to some of the facilities and can sell services to the private unit. The private unit faces reduced overheads and can afford to give the DHA substantial revenue, and still make a profit.

Bioplan have been particularly successful in establishing day-surgery units adjacent to hospital sites. These share various facilities, often giving the NHS access to the beds. As part of the deal, Bioplan guarantee extra revenue to the DHA, partly through the purchase of support services.

Obviously, wearing my private sector hat, I favour such arrangements, but I have a general reservation regarding joint ventures. Rather like sub-contracting services such as catering, managerial freedom is reduced, and rarely do schemes offer sufficient profit for there to be enough to genuinely satisfy both parties — my own view is that 'half a profit' is hardly likely to be worthwhile.

I fear that the motivation on behalf of general managers is not that they have an even-handed approach to such schemes but, rather, they are fairly desperate to raise any revenue, or profit, and even a poor share is better than nothing. There is a serious risk that they are mortgaging their futures in some cases.

Such plans do require Treasury approval, which will be likely to act as a brake on some of the more unconventional proposals. The constraint of the Public Sector Borrowing Requirement will also limit such activity.

Human resources

There are many complaints that the private sector poaches staff from the NHS, and a number of doubts regarding the role of medical staff.

In general terms, the private view is that it is not the NHS which paid to train staff, but rather the tax-payer, and that, in terms of fairness, the private sector finds it hard enough to compete against a free service, without then being blamed for other sins. If, in due course, competition is fairer between the two sides, then I think that the private sector will accept the need to bear the cost of training staff — cynics will even point out that some students are better value than trained staff.

Because of staff shortages, which face both public and private hospitals, many private units are already looking hard at training staff, such as ODAs in operating theatres. Certainly, for nurses, post-basic training is common in the private sector, not only to develop staff, but also as a way to attract and retain staff.

With regard to junior doctors, most private hospitals now have resident medical officers. Unfortunately most such posts are not accredited for training and it is therefore hard to attract good doctors. In London, many private units now contract such services from teaching hospitals and medical schools, and this can work well. The inducement in such recruitment is that such an RMO post can lead to a better chance of obtaining a recognised or good research post.

The role of consultants has typically been the most contentious. Critics argue that NHS consultants spend too much time attending to their private practice. The perception from the private sector is rather that doctors generally work very hard, with long hours, and have a strong sense of loyalty to the NHS. They therefore often more than fulfil their commitment to the NHS, and might even do more if their NHS facilities, such as beds and operating slots, were not limited. No doubt some do abuse their contracts, but I suspect it is more often those who do not do private practice but, rather, spend the rest of the week playing golf.

Some private hospitals have considered the possibility of employing full-time surgeons which might reduce the cost per case of the professional fees. However, the general feeling is that the traditional system of referrals from general practitioner to consultant works well, and that GPs would not happily refer patients to the hospital, or to a doctor who has not proved his quality by obtaining a consultant post.

Incidentally, it is worth bearing in mind that consultant pay within the NHS is poor relative to that of other professions, and there is, in effect a tacit recognition that the consultant will supplement it with private fees. It may be the self-governing Trust hospitals will pay more competitive salaries, but link them to the use of private facilities at the Trust hospital, to the disadvantage of local private hospitals.

Future developments

It is difficult and somewhat dangerous to write this chapter at such a time of change. The Review means that there may be a substantial change in the nature of the NHS, if the details match up to the broad outlines. The creation of the self-governing hospitals will create NHS units which will mimic private units to a considerable extent. Instead of hospitals at two ends of a spectrum, we will have a more continuous range of options.

The separation of funding and provision, if properly done, will create competition within the NHS, and allow private units to compete for the same business. Some observers see this as the first step towards privatisation although the government firmly deny this possibility.

It certainly opens the way towards giving patients vouchers which they could freely exchange at the hospitals of their choice. Such a scheme gives power to the consumers, and would mean that public and private hospitals would all be subjected to common competition and standards. As yet, it is too early to predict how far such a development will go.

The hope must be that there will continue to be a strong NHS along with a thriving private sector service. Not only will they jointly cover the whole spectrum of demand, but, hopefully, spur each other on to higher standards, and a real responsiveness to our customers' demands.

I believe that there is now greater understanding and willingness to co-operate between the two sides, and trust that the Review will result in a friendly and developing relationship, with increasing sharing and trading of health care facilities and services.

Summary

Haydn Cook

The private health-care industry has now reached a state of maturity. After a period of rapid growth it has stabilised, and the time has come to take stock and to look to the future.

Present standards

'Going private' used to be a serious moral issue: times have changed and using a convenient, customer-orientated private hospital is seen to make good sense. Many fears have been expressed as to the nature of the private sector, but what is it really like?

By contrast with the NHS, the private sector is expected to be more commercial, more profit orientated, and, by implication, less caring. In reality, this appears to be not the case. Why is that? The answer is that essentially the same sort of people work in private hospitals as in the NHS hospitals, and the need to care for people tends to rub off on the staff, although most are already part of that self-selecting group of caring people.

Moreover, standards within each industry are driven by customer demands and requirements. Within private health care it is quite clear what patients want, which is excellent care and reasonable value. The consultants support the patients in this view, and lobby for good standards and, similarly, the insurance companies could not approve hospitals which might fall seriously short of an acceptable standard.

Enforcing standards

The system of registration, as described by Paul Ridout (Chapter 7) ensures that there is a reasonable scrutiny of private sector facilities. Accreditation of doctors helps ensure that the hospitals are selective in terms of those practitioners who may have admitting privileges. Obviously the private hospitals cannot, of themselves, enforce a perfect standard with regard to medical users. If society permits underqualified doctors to practise, and peer-review is not effective, then it is hardly reasonable to demand that private hospitals should hold the line. Two factors work in favour of a good actual standard. General practitioners still play a key role in referring patients, and select the right consultant. They will also be loath to refer to anyone who works at a hospital of dubious standard.

Similarly, most hospitals are obliged to be selective in their medical users, since the majority of doctors will boycott hospitals which do not set high standards of accreditation. The Independent Hospitals Association recently published their own guidelines on accreditation, which have been generally accepted as reasonable and practicable. The requirements of insurance companies also naturally enforce good standards. Because of the threat of litigation, hospitals need insurance cover for malpractice and other risks, and the insurers, rightly, seek reassurance that risks are low owing to the achievement of good clinical standards.

However, the above are rather negative expressions of a commitment to good standards. In practice, there are other means of achieving those standards. Most hospitals, for example, document their policies and procedures, along with various implicit or explicit standards. Clinical protocols are part of this, as are health and safety policies.

Improving standards

More importantly, most hospitals and owners believe that good performance in financial terms is linked to a high quality of service. One company at least bases senior staff bonuses partly on achieving financial targets, but the balance is paid if quality targets are achieved. The philosophy is that if the quality standards are achieved, then, given reasonable market conditions, profits will follow. Certainly the manager will have done his best by the company by achieving the quality goals.

A more general study has shown that quality of service determines market share, and that this in turn feeds through to profit. Most health-care companies are now convinced by this argument. As a result there is less competition based on price (prices are matched rather than price-cutting being the priority), and the emphasis is on quality and service. The intention is that both the doctors and the patients will receive an excellent package of clinical and service elements.

Customer power

It is inevitable that, on occasion, we fail to achieve our standards. Within the NHS there is a formal complaints procedure, which is required since the patients have little power as customers. Since the NHS patient does not pay personally, at the time of treatment, he can hardly threaten to take the business elsewhere.

Hospital directors in the private sector, when asked if there is a complaints policy, often respond rather negatively. The reason is that the whole ethic of the private sector is to avoid complaints, and to address the matter immediately if there is a problem. Ultimately, the patient will refuse to pay if there remains a problem, so there is a real incentive to sort matters out!

Patient questionnaires are used to monitor quality, and, again, there is a real need to respond, to ensure future customer satisfaction. Despite the good intentions, inevitably there are occasional formal complaints, and these are investigated. Similarly, once in a while a legal matter arises, normally where a patient feels that he has sustained a significant damage, usually from clinical treatment or lack of it. These are dealt with much as within the NHS, although, when possible, they are resolved locally, as insurance premiums are based both on cases brought to court and on cases notified to the insurer, even if not pursued.

Some cases involve criticism of both hospital and doctor. These are particularly difficult, since the doctor is the hospital's primary customer, and the hospital is therefore reluctant to blame the doctor, and yet will not want to shoulder the whole responsibility.

The above comments relate to the 'micro' level. At the broader level, dissatisfaction with a hospital or home might lead to the health authority taking action. In practice, however, the doctors, as informed customers, will determine on behalf of themselves and their patients, that a particular unit should not be patronised. Competition between units tends to create a self-correcting mechanism, with the unit that loses business being forced to raise standards, or, alternatively change the senior staff or owner.

The future

I believe that there is a strong future for the private sector, although there is much fear that the NHS Review may create some potent competitors. Certainly if they were to 'get their act together' the hospitals which become Trusts could challenge the private hospitals.

However, the existing forces of competition have created strong private sector managers, who are used to responding to challenges. The provision of good quality care and service is part of their skill and expertise, and their priority. For the NHS, their main role will still be the provision of general care, and their private work will still be a minor part of their role. As a result they are unlikely to manage it as effectively as the private-sector managers.

I can foresee, despite the above, that it is likely that new standards and grades of care will evolve. The airlines have moved from First Class and Ordinary Class, to other categories including Business and Charter. Competition from the Trusts is likely to create a new service, based on good clinical care, and reasonable hotel services. If private care currently is 'Five Star', this new grade might be likened to 'Two Star'. No doubt there will be a single room, and a telephone, but it will not compete in all areas.

The private hospitals may have to respond, since, in many ways, competition has driven some standards too high, and something more economic may be acceptable. Certainly the insurance companies will welcome such a move if it makes the cost of the insurance, which funds much health care, more affordable.

Conclusions

The chapters within this book reflect current thinking on many of the issues within private health care. Competition has driven us forward, and helped us to achieve our present standards.

We face continuing challenges to our management abilities, and have to respond and develop accordingly.

Most of us enjoy our work, thrive on the challenges, and grow through our achievements. Little do we know quite what the future will bring, but we are well equipped to meet the unknown. We should congratulate ourselves on what we have built over the last two decades, and look forward with excitement and enthusiasm.

Appendix 1

Guidelines for rating standards for private nursing homes

(Prepared by the Lewisham and North Southwark Health Authority)

1.1   *General/environment*
1.1.1   A friendly and homely atmosphere is maintained.
1.1.2.   Acceptability of environment to patients and staff.
1.1.3.   The Home is clean and free from odours.

1.2.   *Health and safety/fire*
1.2.1.   Presence of handrails on stairs and in corridors, bathrooms and lavatories.
1.2.2.   Fire exits clearly marked and have free access.
1.2.3.   Regular Fire Drills take place for all staff and are recorded.
1.2.4.   Fire fighting equipment is inspected and maintained, as required, and records kept.
1.2.5   Home is well lit.
1.2.6.   All areas are properly and safely heated.

1.3.   *Catering*
1.3.1.   Ethnic minorities' needs are considered in the choice of food.
1.3.2.   Food is attractively served, and in adequate amounts according to appetite.
1.3.3.   Food is served at appropriate temperature.
1.3.4.   Kitchen is clean.
1.3.5.   Kitchen staff are aware of and practise good/hygienic techniques in preparing food.

1.4   *Clinical and general waste*
1.4.1.   Correct methods are used for the disposal of clinical and general waste.

1.5.   *Policies/procedures*
1.5.1.   Written policies/procedures are available.
1.5.2.   Staff are conversant with, and carry out policies/procedures.

1.6   *Brochure*
1.6.1.   A brochure containing details of services provided is available.

1.7.   *Medication*
1.7.1.   Drugs are correctly stored, administered and disposed of.

1.8.   Contracts
1.8.1.   Contract issued to each patient (or relative).

1.9.   Attitude/morale of staff

1.10.   Security
1.10.1. There are facilities for the safe custody and recording of patients' valuables.
1.10.2. There is adequate protection from 'intruders'.

1.11.   Laundry
1.11.1. Provision for laundering of personal clothing on site.
1.11.2   Provision for general (bed linen) laundry.
1.11.3. Provision for foul/infected linen.

2.1   Health care
2.1.1.   Nurse staffing levels are at agreed numbers.
2.1.2.   GP visits regularly and on demand.
2.1.3.   There is a regular access to physiotherapy.
2.1.4.   There are regular checks on teeth, sight and hearing.
2.1.5.   A chiropodist visits regularly.
2.1.6.   Staff training programmes are available and implemented, e.g. lifting and handling techniques.
2.1.7.   There is a programme for promotion of continence.
2.1.8.   Individual care plans are available, up-to-date, and are all corrected, dated and signed.
2.1.9   Patients receive correct medication at the correct time.
2.1.10. Staff have good knowledge of, and carry out procedures correctly, e.g. sterile dressings, procedures for prevention of pressure sores.
2.1.11. There is a functioning Nurse Call System throughout the Home.
2.1.12. Patients are satisfied and happy.
2.1.13   Patients are well-cared for, e.g. hair combed, teeth/mouth clean, mental state, personal clothing.
2.1.14. Equipment/'aids' are available and used.
2.1.15   All available equipment is correctly maintained, e.g. lifts.

3.1   Social and community factors
3.1.1.   Visiting arrangements are flexible.
3.1.2.   Links exist with local churches, voluntary services and schools.
3.1.3.   Patient activities are organised.
3.1.4.   There are facilities/equipment for patients to pursue their own hobbies/interests.

3.1.5. Patients have simple and private access to a telephone.
3.1.6. Evidence of clocks, calendars, up-to-date newspapers and journals to aid orientation.

3.2 Staff
3.2.1. Staff are neat/clean in uniform.
3.2.2. They are welcoming and informative to visitors.
3.2.3. Staff have good knowledge of patients' background and family.
3.2.4. Staff are conversant with the practice and the aims of the Home.
3.2.5. Staff involve patients (where possible) or relatives in planning their own care.

4.1. Personal dignity/identity
4.1.1. There are personal belongings in patients' rooms.
4.1.2. Patients are dressed in their own clothes, including underclothing and footwear.
4.1.3. Patients are wearing their own dentures, and they fit.
4.1.4. Patients have their own toiletries, e.g. flannel, talcum powder.
4.1.5. Rising times and bed times are flexible.
4.1.6. There is a compatible grouping of chairs in communal areas (where possible).
4.1.7. Regular hairdressing service is arranged.

4.2. Meals
4.2.1. There is a varied menu of the patient's choice.
4.2.2. Meals are nutritious.
4.2.3. Ethnic and religious needs are accommodated.

4.3. Privacy
4.3.1. There is privacy for patients to talk to their visitors.
4.3.2. Catheter Drainage Bags are concealed.
4.3.3. Personal mirrors are available.
4.3.4. Bathing, washing, toiletting is undertaken with privacy.

4.4. Independence
4.4.1. The preferred mode of address is accorded to each patient.
4.4.2. Each patient controls his/her own money where possible or appropriate.
4.4.3. Patients are given both time and essential equipment to feed themselves.
4.4.4. There is a designated area where patients may smoke, which is no less warm and attractive than other areas in the Home.
4.4.5. Patients are allowed alcohol (unprescribed).

Appendix 2

The use of psychometric tests in human-resource decision-making

Peter Naylor*

The UK labour market is changing, more is known about some of the personal variables that seem to promote work effectiveness and employees are more valued as people. When making decisions affecting people at work, these factors and keener global competition are causing more and more employers to reappraise the personal criteria used and the basis for evaluating them. It has and will become even more necessary for these decisions to be, and to be seen as fair, reliable and practicable. This is certainly as true in the medicare field as in other sectors of the economy, if not more so.

These factors seem to be increasing the use of psychometric or psychological tests by UK employers including some in medicare. Many seem to find these to be a useful adjunct to the ever popular but notoriously unreliable selection interview. Others use them in assessment centres for career management and training needs assessment and in counselling.

A wide range of tests exist. Many but by no means all, have been designed and validated in the US, like the 16 PF, the California Personality Inventory and the Myers Briggs Type Indicator. Amongst those which have been developed in the UK, are the Occupational Personality Questionnaire, the Eysenck Personality Profile and the Graduate and Management Assessment Battery.

They embrace inventories, indicators and questionnaires. All aim to distinguish one person's characteristics and abilities from those of another before becoming, or once they have become, an employee. These are tests of: personality; interests; attainment; general intelligence; special aptitude or ability.

It is not practicable to describe the many tests which are available in each of the categories listed. Readers are referred elsewhere to a series of brief descriptions which illustrate the types of tests that are available from the huge number which have been devised (Toplis, Dulewicz and Fletcher, 1987). When considering their use, however, a number of things have to be done and considered.

---

*Peter Naylor is Chairman of Catalysis Ltd

The first is to establish what sorts of factors seem to be important determinants affecting an individual's job performance. Usually and desirably this means undertaking job analysis, identifying important personal variables and relating these to an assessment of individual performance. Once a representative sample of employees has been studied in this way and data about them collected, these data have to be analysed statistically to establish the nature, degree and significance of any one variable with that of their assessed performance or other quantitative and qualitative measures of the output from their work.

If there do appear to be identifiable personal characteristics and abilities that seem to relate to or affect these performance criteria, the second stage is to establish whether or not reliable, valid and validated tests are available which do assess them. Further analytical work, research and discussion will be necessary; usually to make sure that the chosen tests do what you want them to do and are suitable, reliable, easy to obtain, update and administer in the working environment and within the process(es) for which they are intended to be used.

It is then necessary to determine at what stage in a procedure the tests are to be used, by whom and in association with what other techniques. This last point is particularly important since it is highly undesirable to rely only on one technique or test, particularly when making decisions on selection and promotion.

Adequate and responsible use and interpretation of psychometric tests depends on three important conditions being satisfied. First, the interpreter must be knowledgeable about the general design principles of tests and their measurement and suitably qualified to use them.

Secondly, tests must not be interpreted in isolation. The results must be interpreted in a context. This comprises what is already known about the individual and the organisational environment in which he does or may work. Factors such as education, intelligence, work and life experience, cultural and ethnic variables and the reasons why tests are being used, will and should also affect the ways in which test results are interpreted.

Thirdly, that the test or tests must be available to appropriately qualified users from a reputable supplier.

Suppliers must be able and willing to supply and update information on the reliability, validity, acceptability, effectiveness, normative data, bias and availability of tests. If any of this information is not available about a test, it should not be used.

There are no circumstances where 'home made' tests or 'second hand' versions of established tests should be used by people who are not suitably qualified. The skills and professionalism of a trained psychometrician are vital to do the range of complex work necessary before any test is used.

Most of the psychometric instruments in popular use are based on a self-report format. In other words, the candidates themselves decide in what ways they answer the questions posed in an inventory. Thus, test designers are and have to be aware of the need to question the validity of what respondents say of themselves. Some candidates may try to put themselves in a favourable light, others in a less favourable one and a few may respond randomly and haphazardly or even carelessly.

Many of the better known and well validated tests are designed so that the interpreter can assess whether or not any of these ways of answering have been used. This information is then used to assess whether or not their extent is such that it means that the overall response an individual makes to a questionnaire is unreliable or invalid. When choosing tests, this design feature and its importance must be borne in mind.

When tests are used to make employment decisions, they should be scored and interpreted only by suitably trained and qualified people. It is best for their assessments of test results to be in writing (Davey and Harris, 1982, give a useful format). It is essential as well as being self-evident, that the assessments must be prepared by comparing the individual's test results to the criteria that have been identified as essential or desirable for acceptable performance, in the way outlined earlier.

Whenever tests are used to guide either the selection or the rejection of candidates, particular care must be taken to avoid discriminating against people unfairly or unlawfully. This is of course quite apart from, and in addition to, the general need to do so in accordance with the relevant laws. The Commission for Racial Equality, the Equal Opportunities Commission, the Institute of Personnel Management (IPM) and the British Psychological Society can be called upon to give reliable, useful, practical and proven and expert advice about this specific aspect of testing and on recruitment and selection in general. They will also give guidance about the steps that must be taken to avoid using tests in an unfair or in an unlawful manner (see end of chapter).

The IPM has published three codes (on Equal Opportunities, on Occupational Testing and on Recruitment) and a book *Psychological Testing — a practical guide for employers* which are essential reading for those using or contemplating the use of tests.

If computers are to be used to administer and to store data associated with psychometric tests, the provisions of the Data Protection Act 1984 must be followed and candidates must be aware of this and have access to the data about them which are held on a computer (see also the IPM code on Employee Data).

There are issues of confidentiality, ethics, administration, training of the staff involved, initial briefing of candidates and feeding back of test results to them. These are all of great importance. Each needs to be considered most carefully, often by calling on outside expert advice, before deciding to use tests in the recruitment or in any of the other processes affecting applicants or employees.

One way of clarifying an organisation's approach, or rather the approach of influential groups of people in an organisation, to these and to more general issues of using tests is to draw up a policy and a set of guidelines that will govern their introduction and continued use. Indeed, some would urge that this is an important first step. Such a document can be used to stimulate discussion and broad agreement about the ethical, legal and practical issues and benefits of using tests. This should lead to the adoption and publication of an agreed policy and a set of guidelines that are to be followed by those involved in their application and interpretation.

Another is to let the key people see the instruments that could be used, to encourage them to complete them and to receive feedback. This can remove some of the mystery and reduce some of the anxiety that people sometimes associate with tests and which can prevent their use.

Feedback should be offered to those candidates or employees who complete tests. It is generally useful and well received. It does need to be carried out with care and sensitivity to the needs of the candidates. It may present difficulties when time and other resources are in short supply. This may be so especially when dealing with external candidates.

Many UK and US psychometricians are bound by professional codes to ensure that they give adequate orientation and information to candidates before and after test administration. This allows the test to be set in an appropriate context along with other relevant factors. Some UK and many US qualifying courses, designed for users to administer a particular test, provide training in the management of feedback.

Once the preliminary studies have been undertaken, tests chosen, decisions taken about how, when, where, by whom and for what purpose(s) tests are to be used, it is all too easy to sit back and think: 'Well, that's another job off the "to do" list!' To do so would be as mistaken as it would be irresponsible. As the IPM Code on Occupational Testing reminds us: 'Once a test has been introduced and is in use, it is essential to continue to monitor its effectiveness...'.

Thus vigilance is required to ensure that:

• standards are upheld;

• the test still meets a need;

• inappropriate decisions are not being made;

• unfair discrimination is being avoided;

• monitoring of the results takes place regularly;

• up-to-date versions of the test are being used;

• up-to-date norms are being used;

• the interpretations being made are still valid;

• the test still gives value for money;

• the test results in effective placement and promotion decisions;

• policies and guidelines are up-to-date, relevant and being followed.

If psychometric tests are to yield the benefits of which they are capable, like any other aid to the decisions which managers and others have to make about people, they need skilful, informed, responsible and careful management. When this is done they can indeed enhance the quality of decisions affecting people and help to make their placement in jobs a more certain process and a more satisfying experience. There are clear economic, social and personal advantages to be gained from their appropriate and responsible use.

Further information

The following can be contacted for more details:

Institute of Personnel Management, IPM House, Camp Road, Wimbledon, SW19 4UX.

The British Psychological Society, St Andrews House, 48 Princess Road East, Leicester LE1 7DR.

The Commission for Racial Equality, Elliot House, 10/12 Allington Street, London SW1E 5EN.

The Equal Opportunities Commission, Overseas House, Quay Street, Manchester M3 3HN.

Further reading and references

Anastasi A 1988 *Psychological testing*, 6th edn. Macmillan, New York

Davey DM, Harris M 1982 *Judging people*. McGraw Hill

Pearn MA, Kandola RS, Mottram RD 1987 *Selection testing and sex bias*. Equal Opportunities Commission

Robson C *Experiment, design and statistics in psychology*. Penguin Books

Toplis J, Dulewicz V, Fetcher C *Psychological testing*. IPM

Tyler LE, Walsh WB 1979 *Tests and measurement*. Prentice-Hall